FOOD ALLERGY CONQUEROR

Ollie's OIT Story

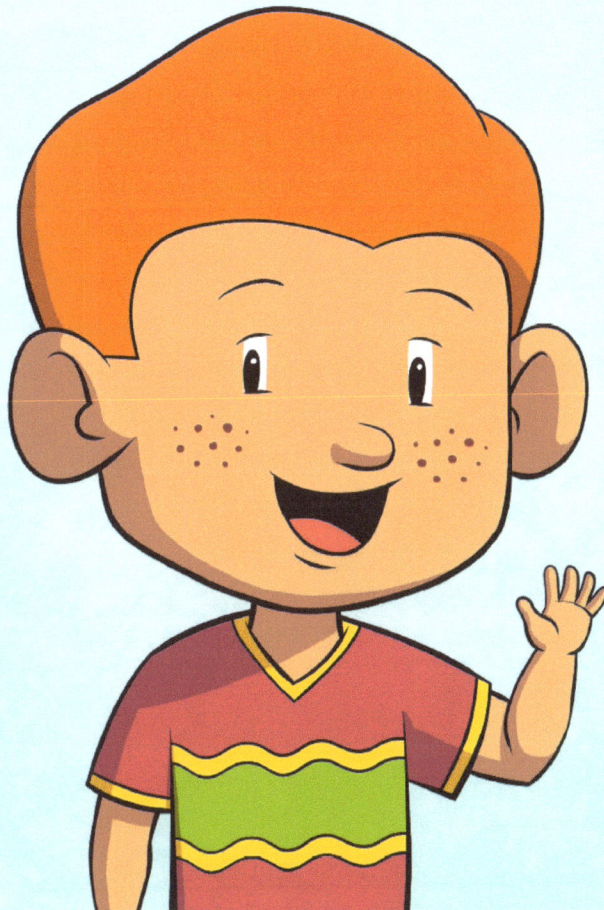

by George W. Browne, M.D.

with Jennifer Browne

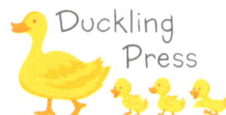

Duckling Press

DEDICATION

To Richard Wasserman, M.D., Ph.D.

And his brave staff, for pioneering this process

And to all of our patients and families

Past, Present, and Future

Published by Duckling Press.

For additional copies or special discounts for bulk purchases as well as booking George W. Browne, M.D. to speak at your event, please email support@ducklingpress.com.

Duckling Press

www.DucklingPress.com

Cover & Interior design by Orange Brain Studio
Illustrations by Marketing Flix
Photography by Caitlin Cannon
Editing by Alyssa Rabins
Composition by Accelerate Media Partners, LLC
ISBN: 978-1-7360895-3-8
HEALTH & FITNESS / Allergies
Printed in the United States of America

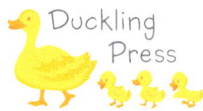

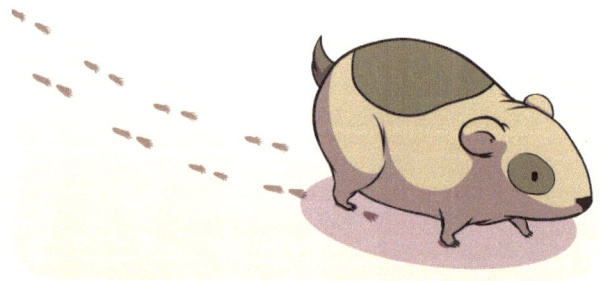

FOREWORD

I first heard about oral immunotherapy (OIT) for food allergy from Dr. Lyndon Mansfield almost 15 years ago. He told me that he had successfully treated a few peanut allergy patients and generously sent me his treatment plans from which I developed our first Dallas Food Allergy Center protocols. I modeled our treatment after allergen immunotherapy (allergy shots). OIT involves retraining (desensitizing) the allergy system by exposing the patient to very tiny, gradually increasing doses of the problem food. Over the past twelve years we have treated more than 850 patients, more than 80% of whom are now able to eat the food to which they had previously reacted. We have also shared our treatment protocols with more than 150 board-certified allergists/immunologists around the world.

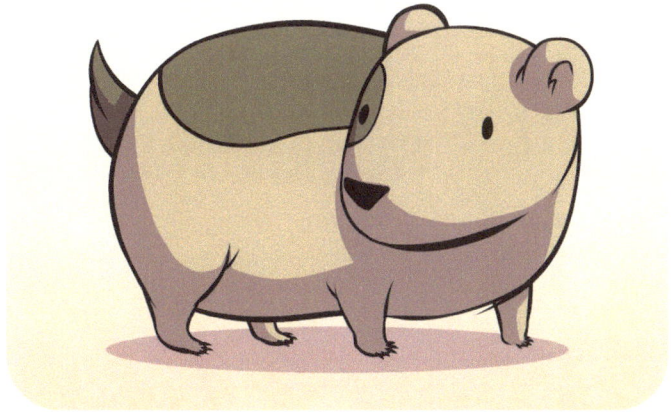

Treating food allergies has been the most rewarding thing I have done in more than 40 years as a physician. Over and over again, families have told me that I have changed their lives for the better.

The Brownes have created a lovely book that captures the hopes, fears, and joys of OIT through the eyes of a child with peanut allergy. The beautifully illustrated tale traces Ollie's journey from the bullied food-allergy kid to a friend able to share a candy bar. This book will help children and parents alike as they begin their own OIT journey with the help of dedicated clinicians, like Dr. George Browne, to guide their way.

Sincerely,

Richard L. Wasserman, M.D., Ph.D.
Medical Director of Pediatric Allergy and Immunology at Medical City Children's Hospital
Director of the Dallas Food Allergy Center

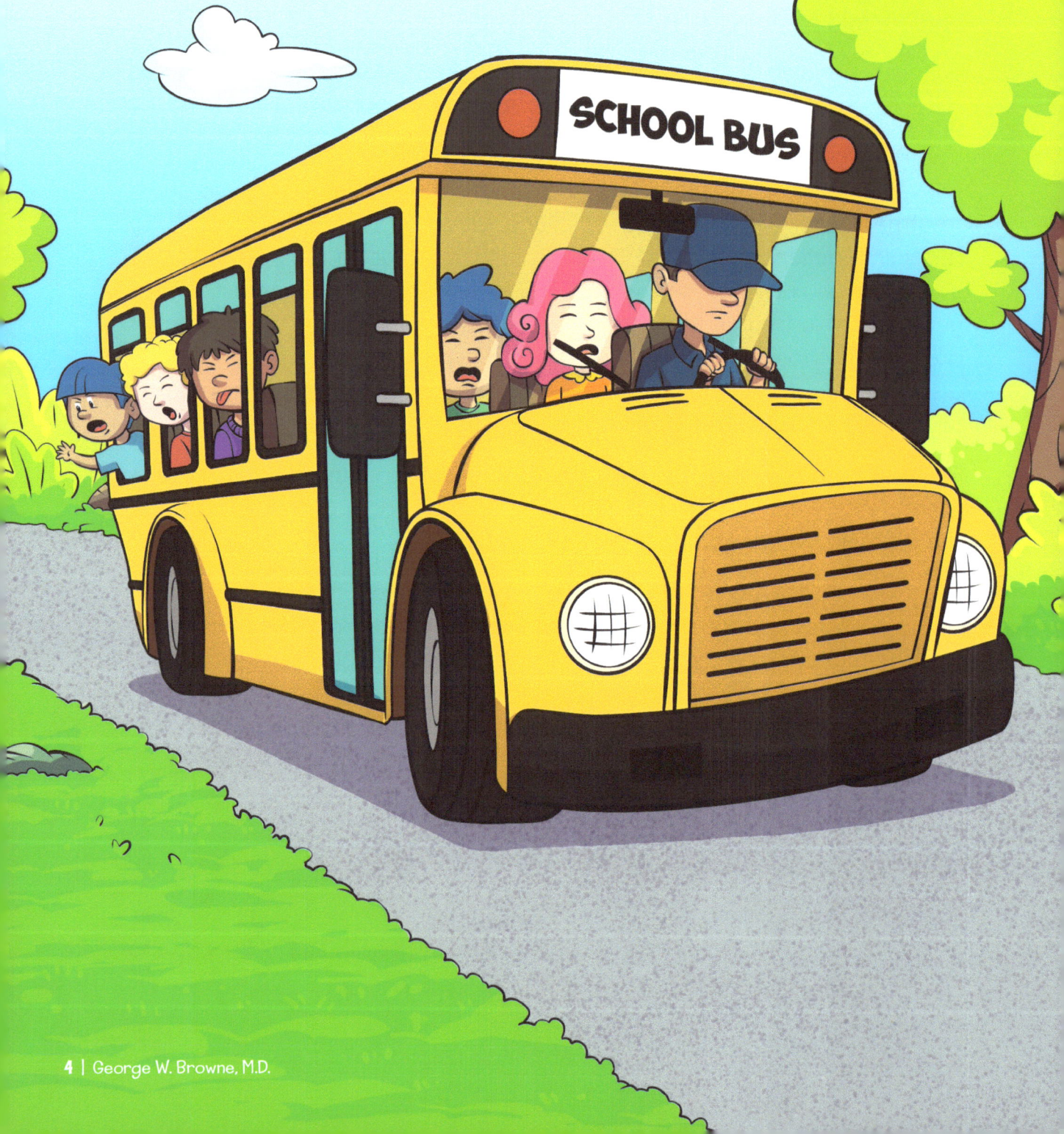

PEANUTS! PEANUTS!
OLLIE'S SCARED OF PEANUTS!

I raced into the house, slamming the door behind me.

"Shh!" Mom hissed. "You'll wake Ethan." My little brother was asleep on the couch.

"Ugh!" I grumbled as I stomped to my room.

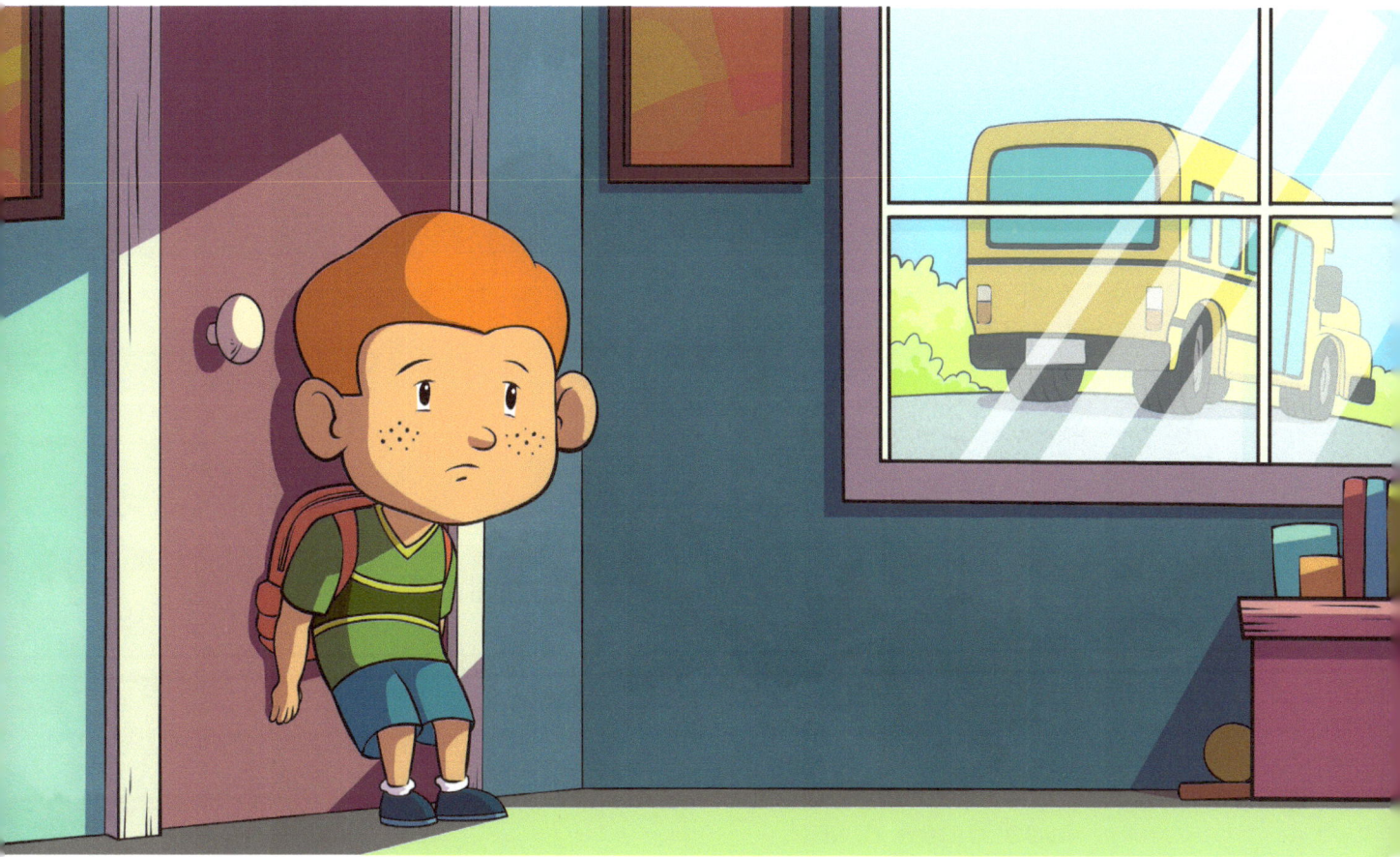

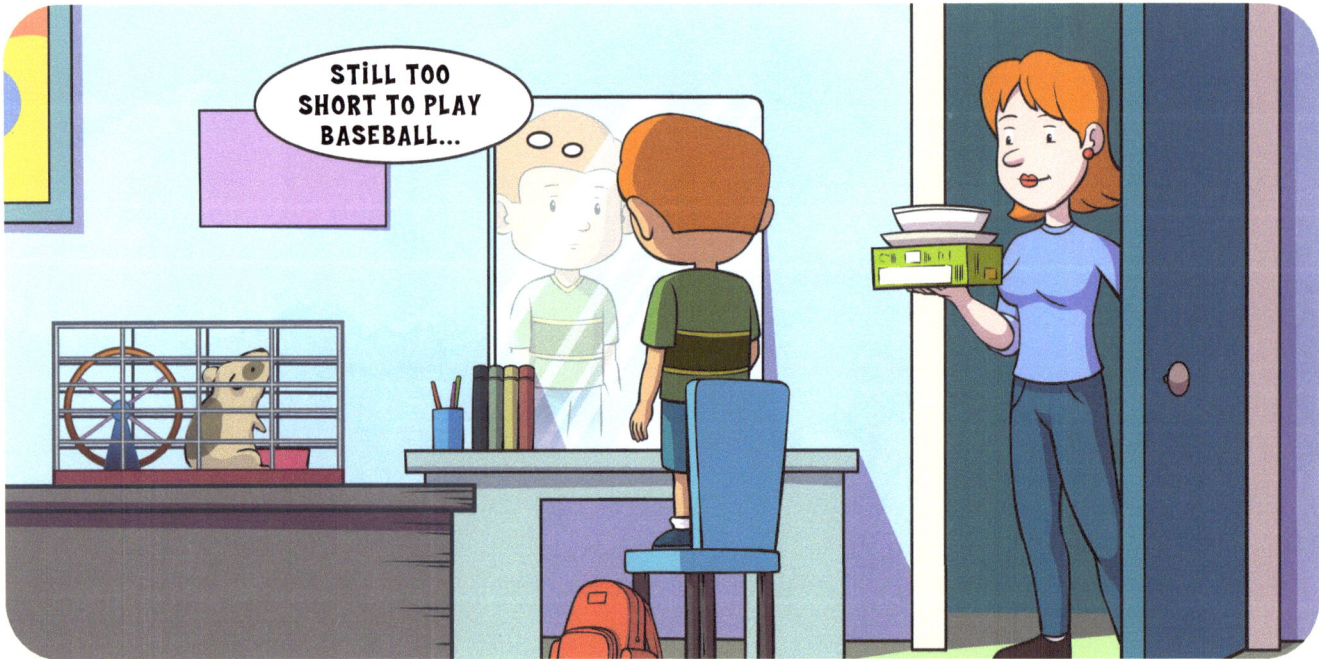

As I dropped my backpack, Mom pushed open the door. She was balancing a tower in one hand—a small bowl, on top of a plate of apple slices, on top of a box.

"How was school?" she asked.

"Mffuugt," I answered, through a mouthful of apple.

"Get dressed for tae kwon do. We need to leave in 30 minutes," Mom said distractedly.

She handed me the box as she left. It was hamster food, a new brand.

I guessed Mom was in a hurry. I figured she didn't need to hear about my bad day now.

I grabbed another slice of apple and dipped it in the sunflower seed butter.

I was starving. I had been too scared to eat lunch. The older boys had wiped their peanut butter hands all over my table on purpose.

I shoved the piece of apple into my mouth.

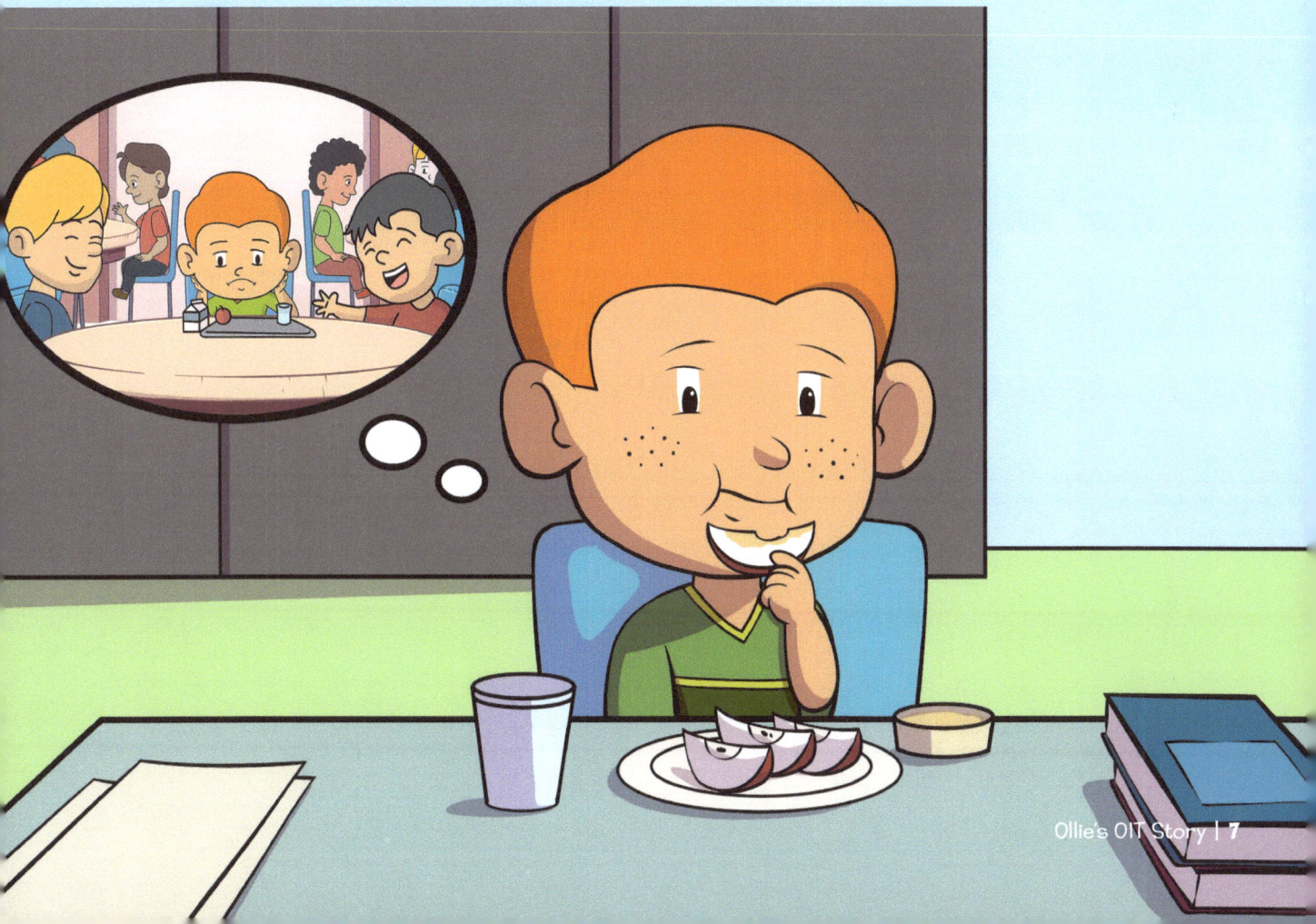

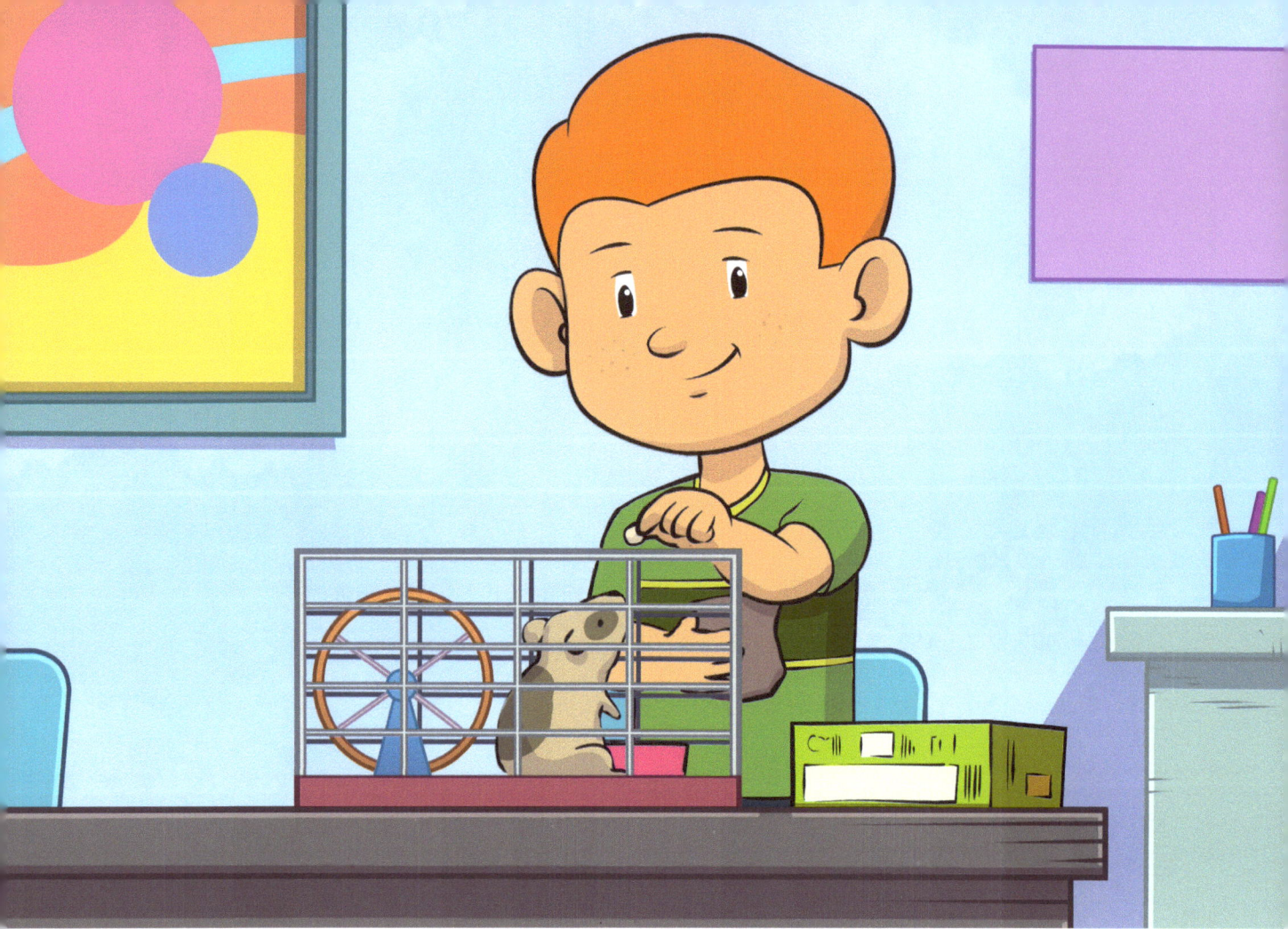

I thought my hamster, Kayson, must be hungry too.

I poured some of the new food into my hand. It was much more colorful than the pellets we usually got.

I put my hand into Kayson's cage and held it very still. He sniffed at it, then greedily grabbed piece after piece and shoved them into his bulging cheeks. His little paws tickled.

I dumped the rest into his bowl and latched the door shut.

I quickly finished off my own snack, licking the sticky dip off my fingers.

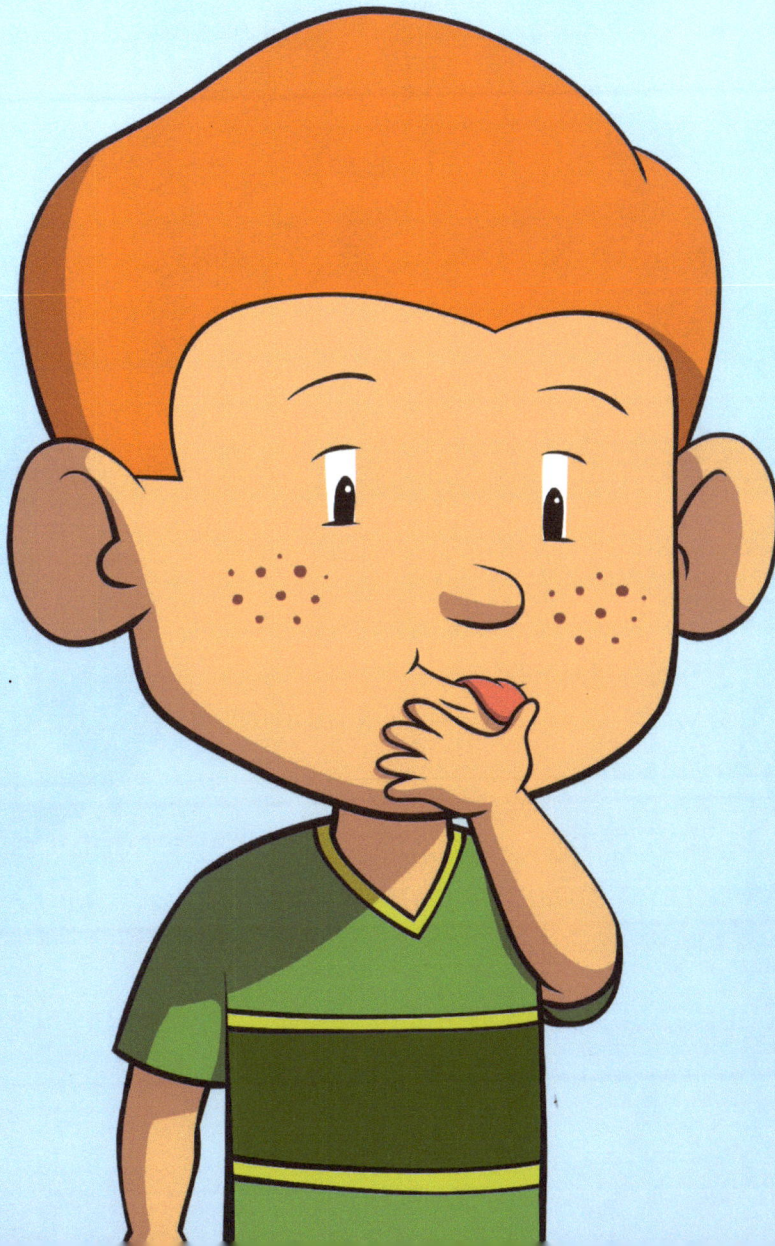

Hmm. My lips felt all tingly. I got out my uniform, but I just couldn't put it on.

It was hard to breathe and I felt a little dizzy. I lay on my bed. Suddenly, I threw up.

"Mom!" I yelped. It squeaked out, kind of hoarse sounding.

She came running and started asking me questions.

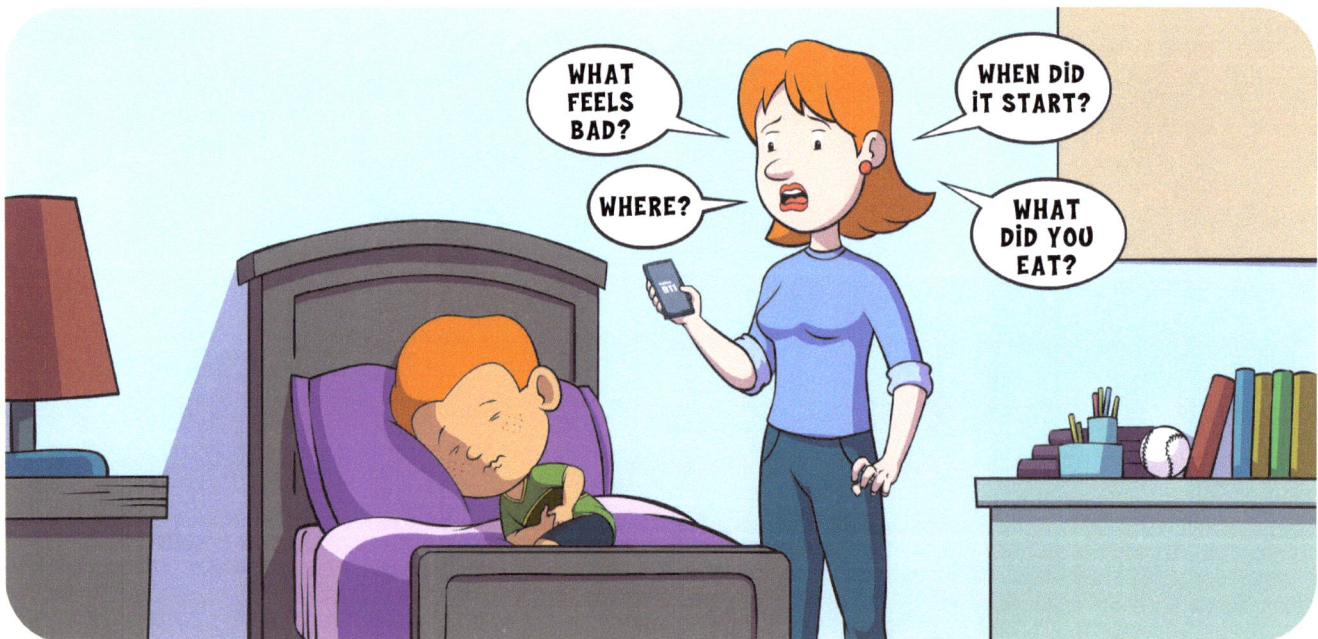

"Just what you gave me," I mumbled. "And I fed Kayson."

"Oh, no!" Things seemed a bit blurry except for the scared look on her face before she ran for my emergency shot.

It hurt, but I barely noticed. Mom called 911.

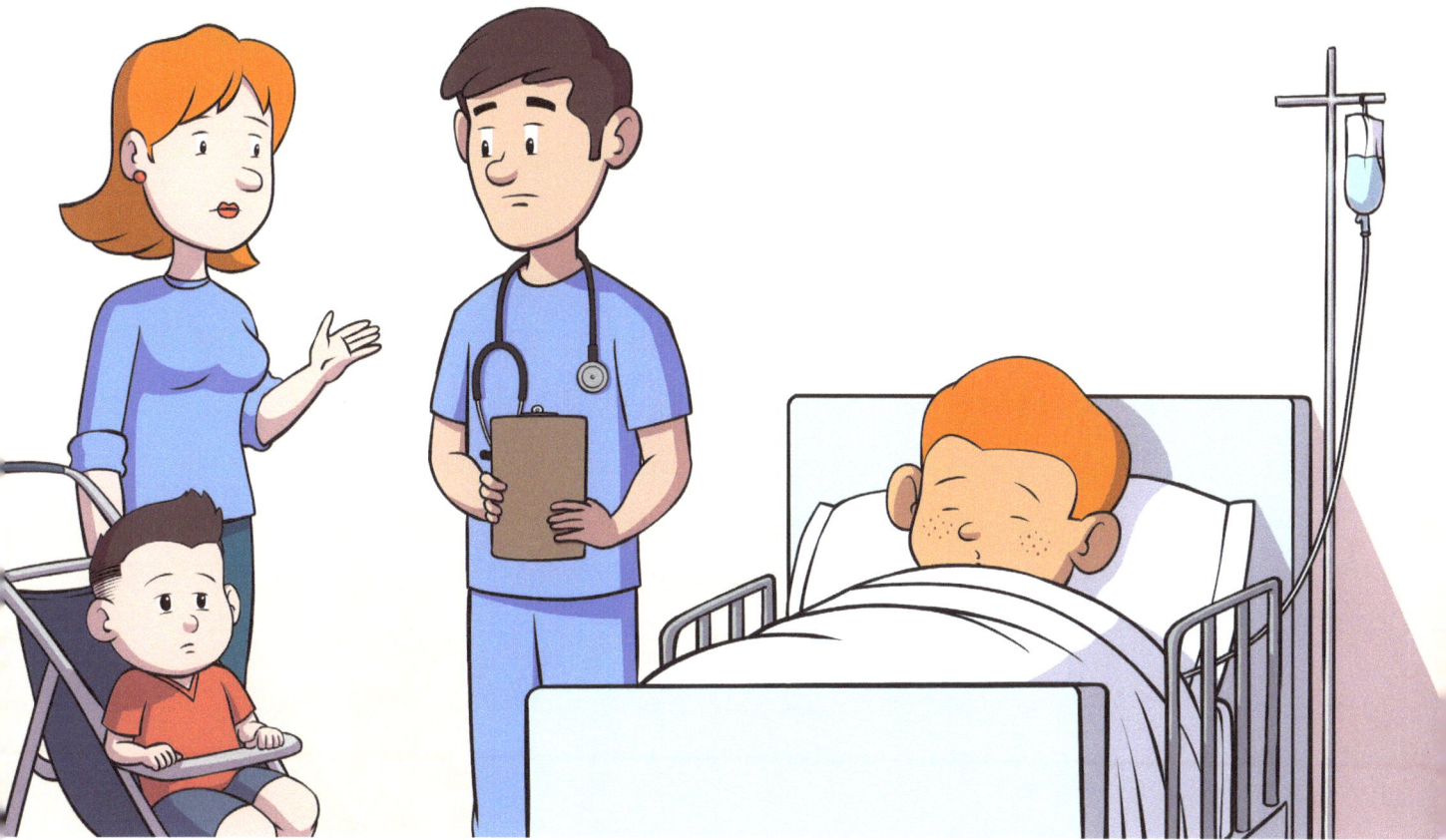

We were at the emergency room for a really long time. A bunch of doctors and nurses checked me over, all asking questions.

They asked us what I had eaten about 50 times, then read and re-read the ingredients on the box of hamster food. It said it could have traces of peanut in it. They decided some must've stuck to my fingers and I ate it.

They sent me home after they were sure I was out of danger.

It was too late to go to tae kwon do.

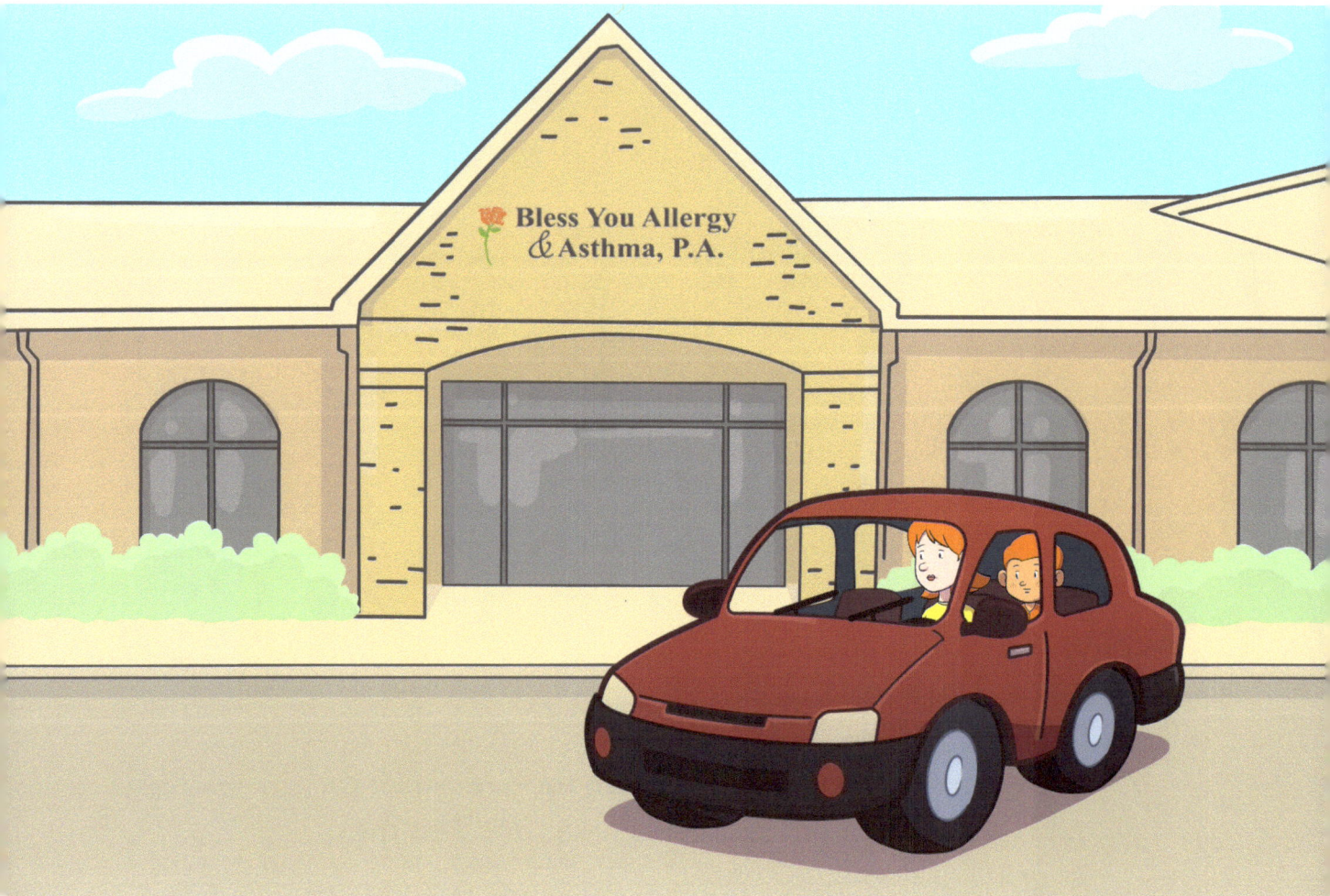

The next afternoon, Mom took me to a new allergist's office. The hospital had recommended we check out a different treatment for allergies like mine. I didn't want to go.

"Allergists," I reminded Mom, "can't change anything."

"Dr. Browne helps kids with food allergies by doing something called oral immunotherapy—which is hard to say!" she chuckled. "The nurse just calls it OIT, so I guess we can too."

The waiting room had cool stuff at least, not just baby toys and grown-up magazines.

The lady behind the desk noticed my baseball T-shirt right away. All the people working there were wearing baseball clothes! I guess they really get into the playoffs around here.

I sat in a chair thinking about my favorite team. When my parents took me to see my first game at the stadium, I started getting itchy because there were so many people eating peanuts around us. We had to leave.

Someone was calling me. It was my turn.

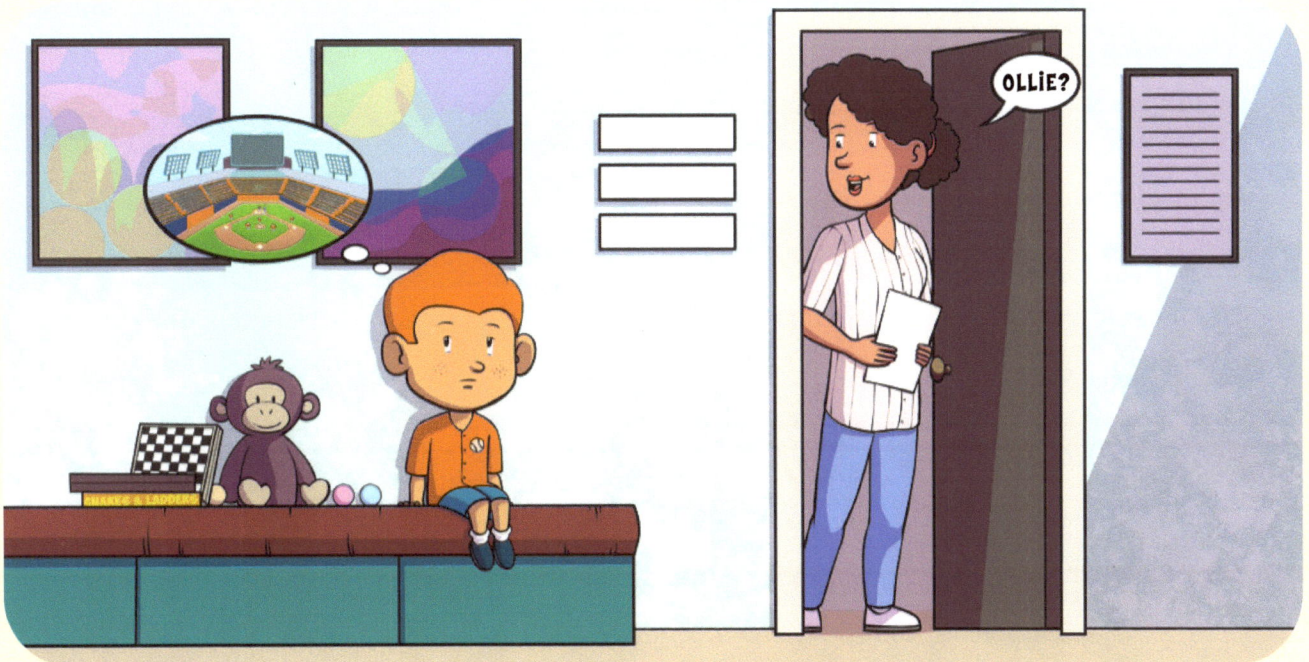

Dr. Browne shook my hand, wearing a huge smile and a blue jersey.

"I'm going to play professional baseball one day," I told him. He said he had a little boy at home who loved sports too.

We had to tell Dr. Browne the whole story of my peanut allergy. He told me I was a really brave kid and said he could help me fix my allergy. He invited my family to come to an information night to hear him and a mom speak about OIT.

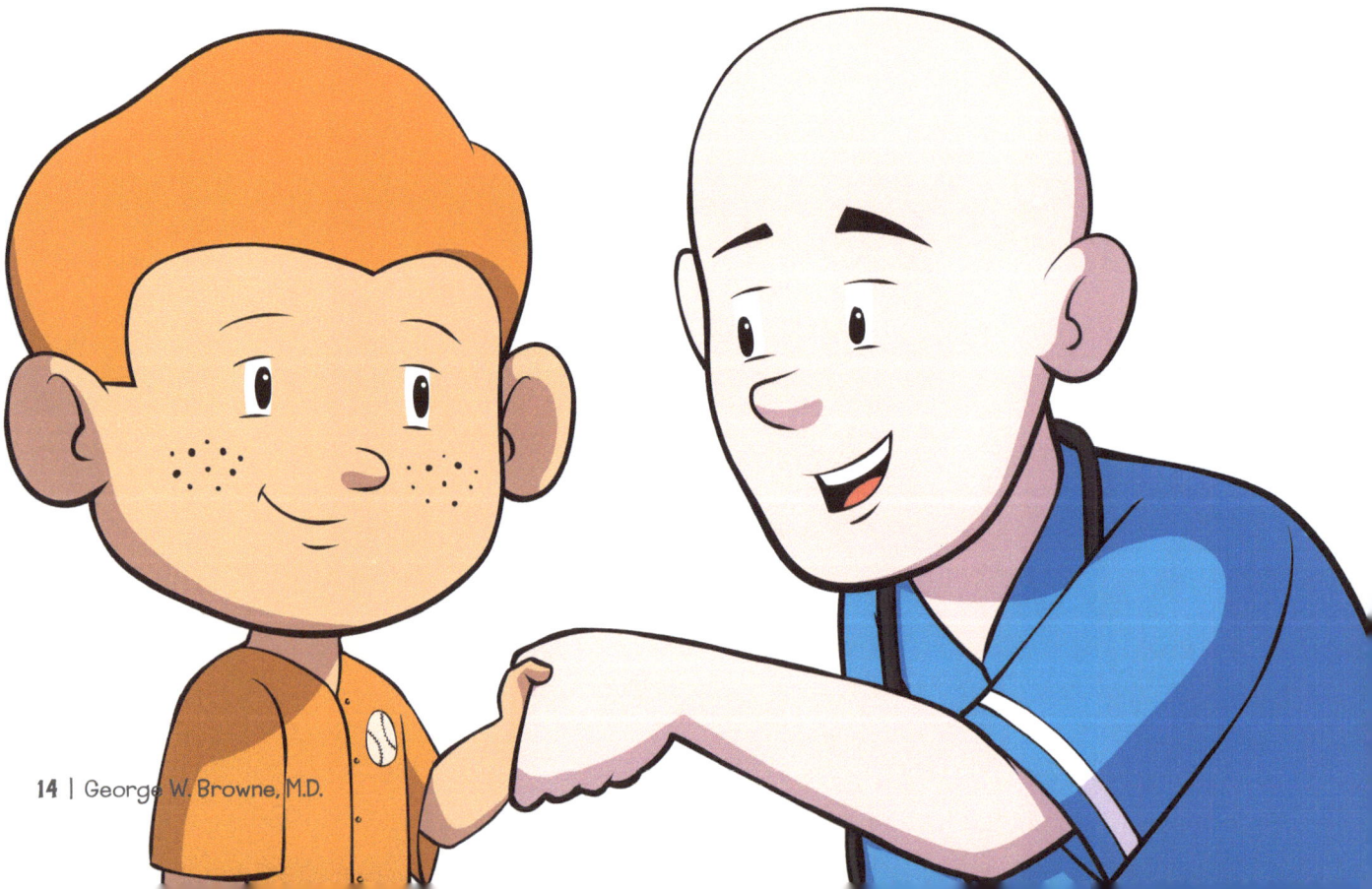

"Ollie," Dr. Browne asked, "if you could eat peanuts, what would your dream food be?"

I paused. I had never thought a lot about actually eating them. Then I got an idea—my dad's favorite candy!

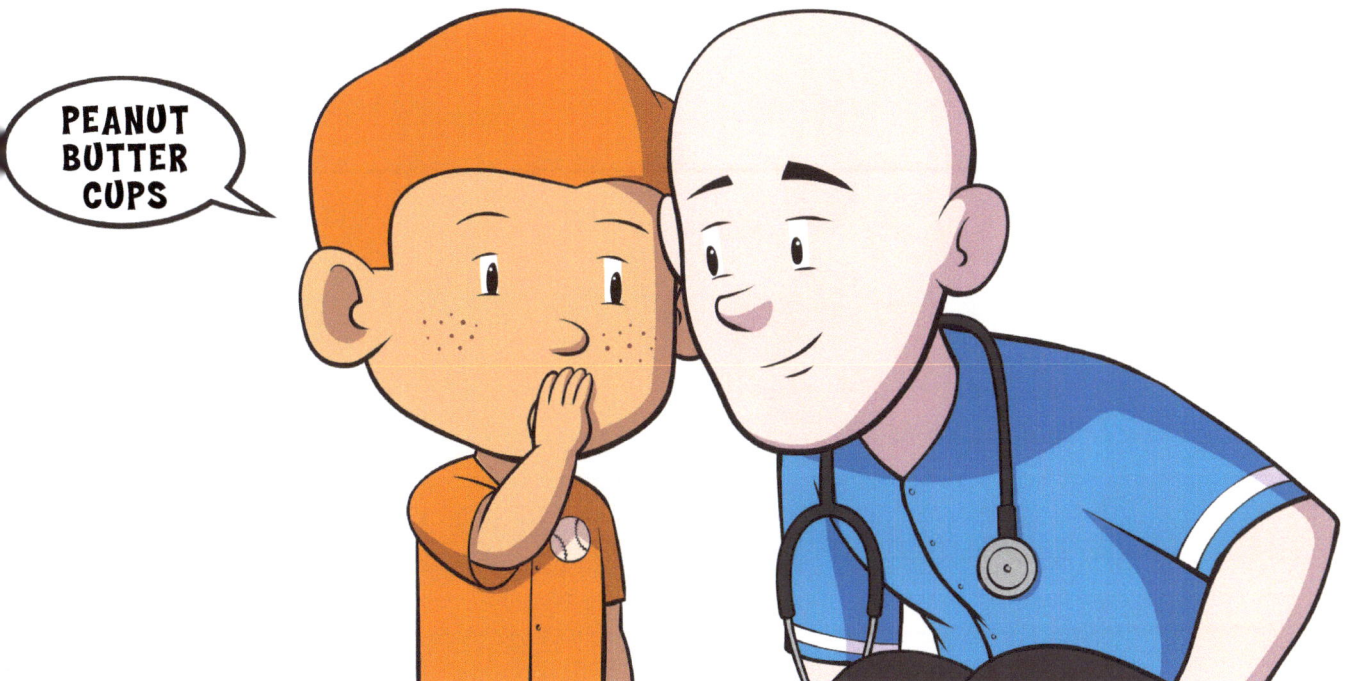

PEANUT BUTTER CUPS

"Those are one of my favorites too," he chuckled.
"Tell you what.
When you are done, we will eat some together."

"All right!" I agreed, "And my dad too?"

"That's a deal."

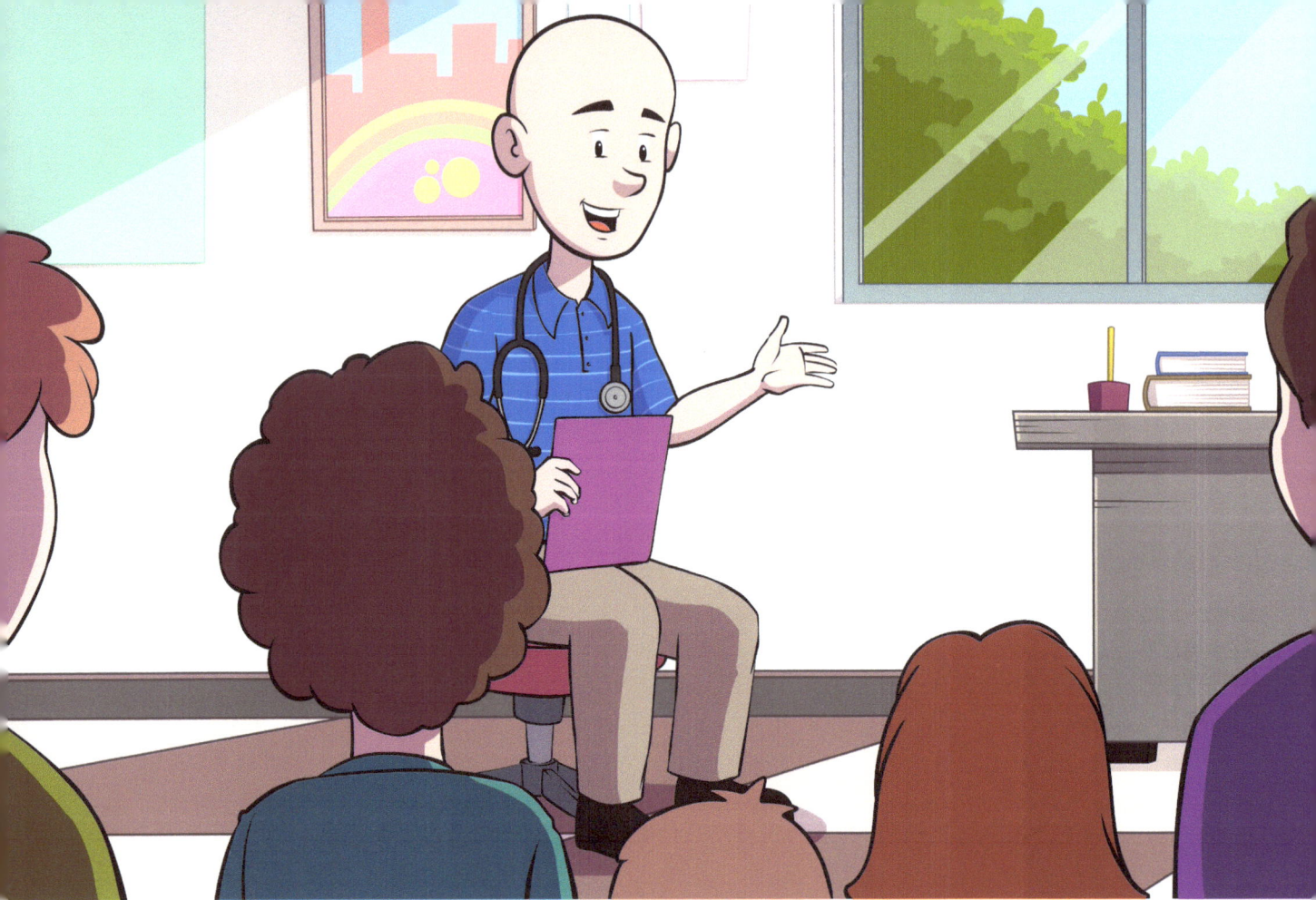

A few weeks later, we were back at the office for the OIT information night.

There were kids there with lots of different kinds of food allergies—wheat, dairy, egg, soy, and all kinds of nuts too. I learned that Dr. Browne can help them all!

If I joined the OIT program, I'd have to drink some juice with tiny bits of peanut in it every day for a few months. They'd give me more and more as my body got used to it.

After that, I would have to eat peanuts every day to keep my body used to them—but I'd be safe.

A girl named Sara, who did OIT for her dairy allergy, told us about how she can have ice cream now and macaroni and cheese—without getting sick!

Her mom talked about how nice it is to not have to read all the labels and watch everything Sara eats.

Her dad also said that their grocery bill has gone down because they don't have to buy special food anymore. I heard my dad chuckle.

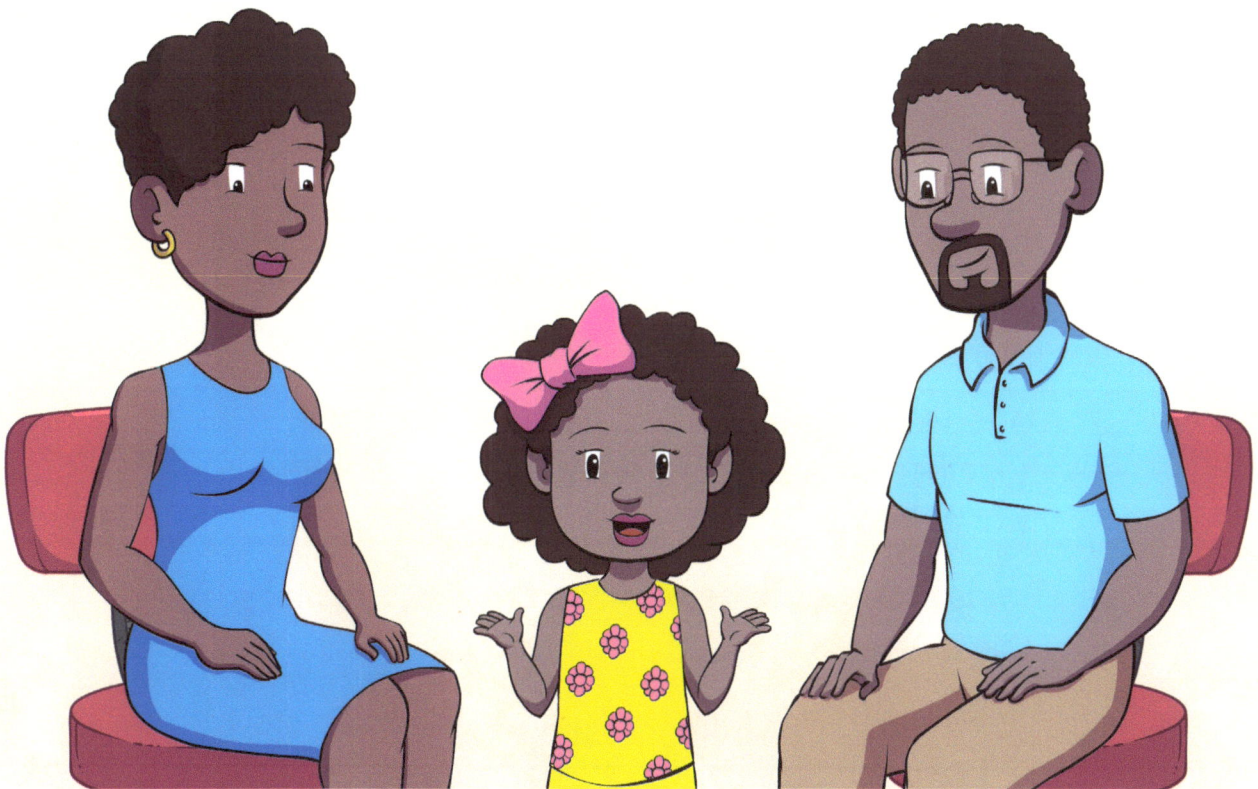

Before we left, Dr. Browne told us that we must never try to do this on our own—no matter how excited we are to get started. We need a doctor watching us every step of the way to make sure we're safe.

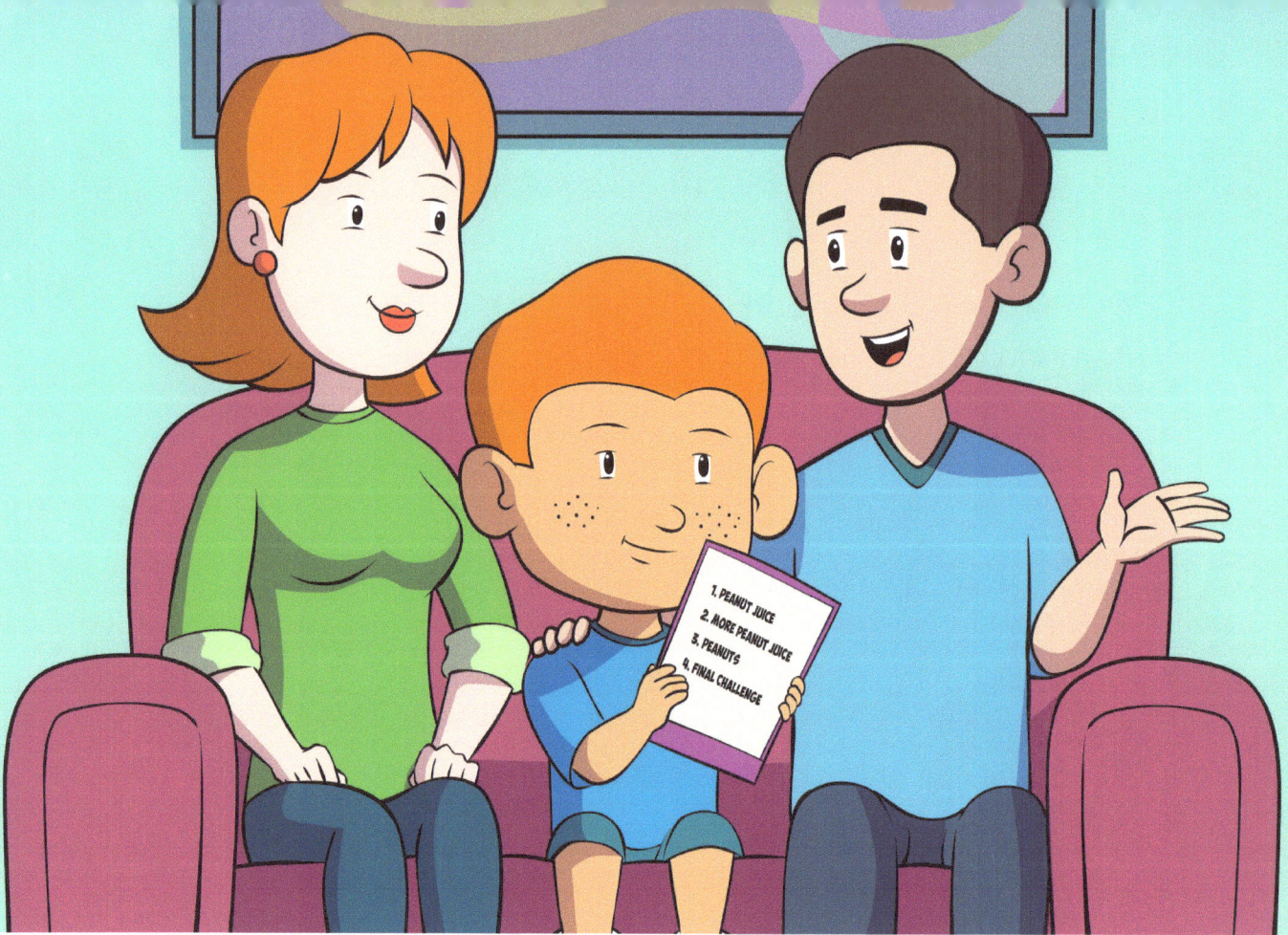

Afterward, Mom and Dad did a lot of talking together and asked me what I thought. I definitely wanted to do it.

I was pretty sure the other parents had convinced them. At least, I hoped they had.

A few days later, they finally decided I could start OIT and scheduled my first appointment.

I started to have dreams about going to baseball games and eating boxes full of peanuts.

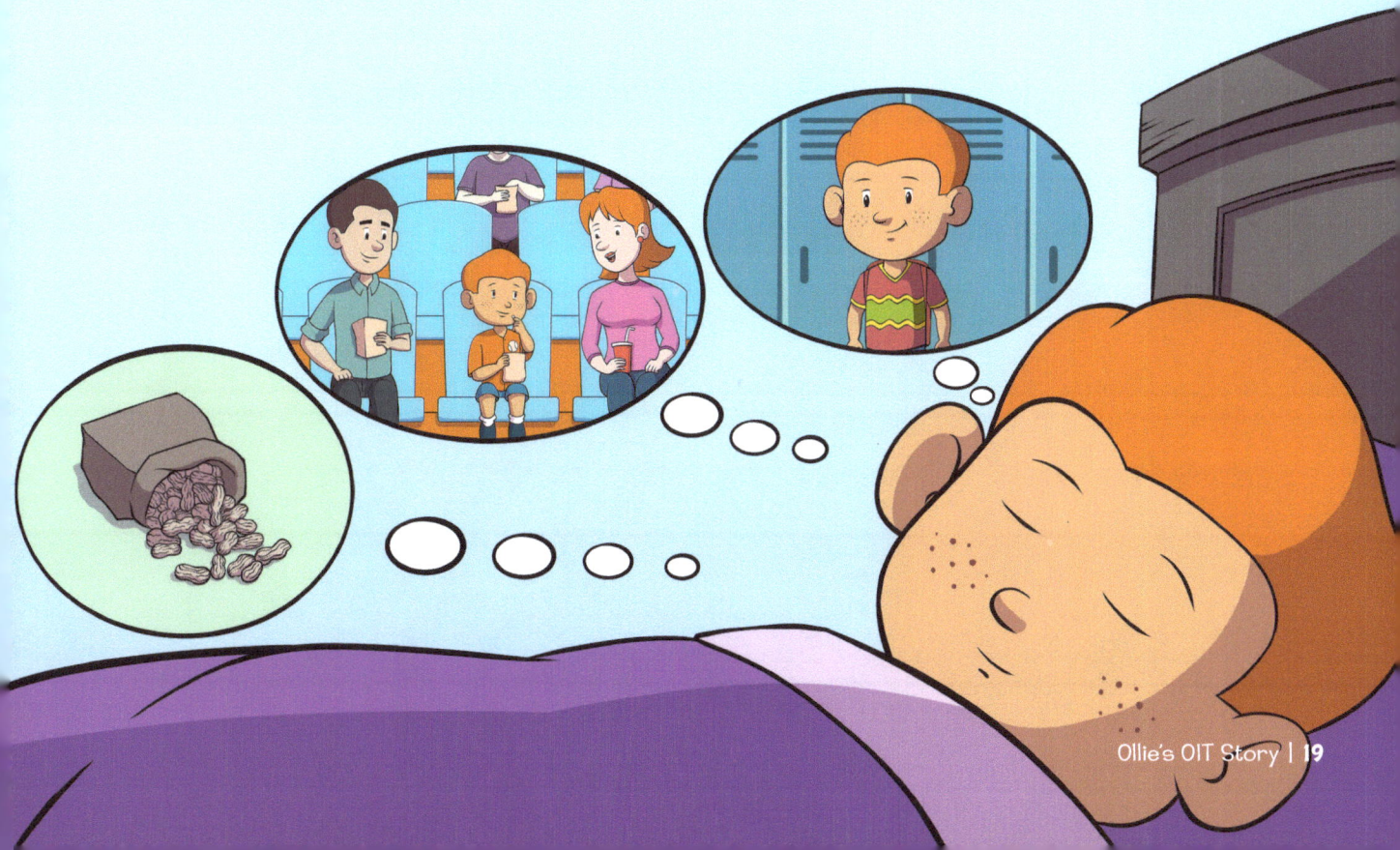

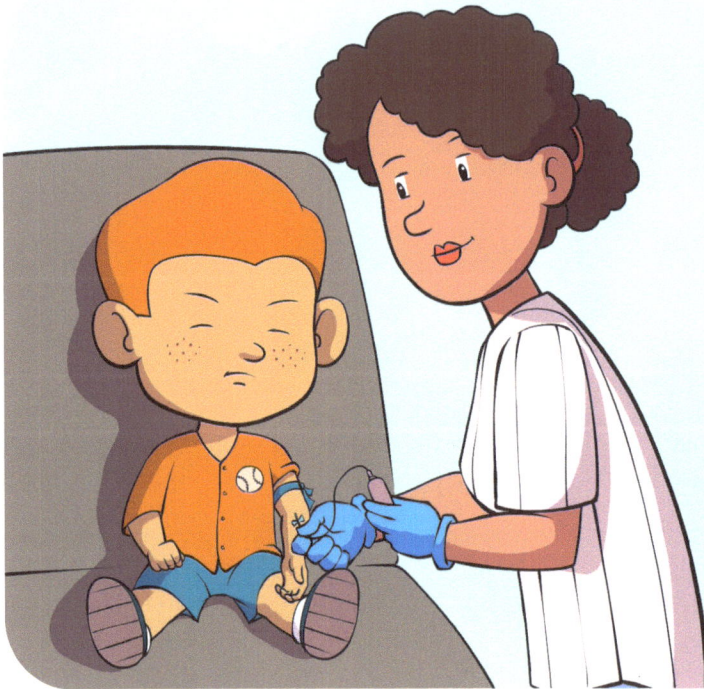

First, I had to go and get some blood taken out of my arm. It hurt when the needle went in, but I just shut my eyes and thought about going to friends' houses and not having to ask about everything I ate.

Then I had a skin test. The nurses pricked my skin with tiny bits of different foods. The spot where they were testing for peanut made a huge, red bump. It didn't hurt much, but it itched like crazy! None of my other pricks got itchy at all.

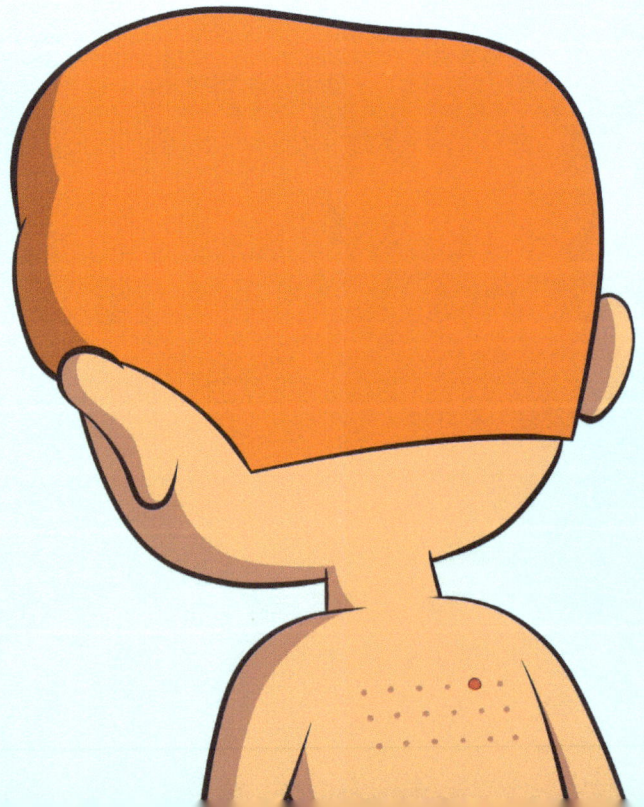

Today I was starting OIT and I felt pretty bouncy inside. Dr. Browne checked on me, and a nurse named Rose came in with a dose of purple juice. She reminded me that it had a teeny, tiny bit of peanut in it. She said I might have a reaction, but they would all be there to stop it if it happened.

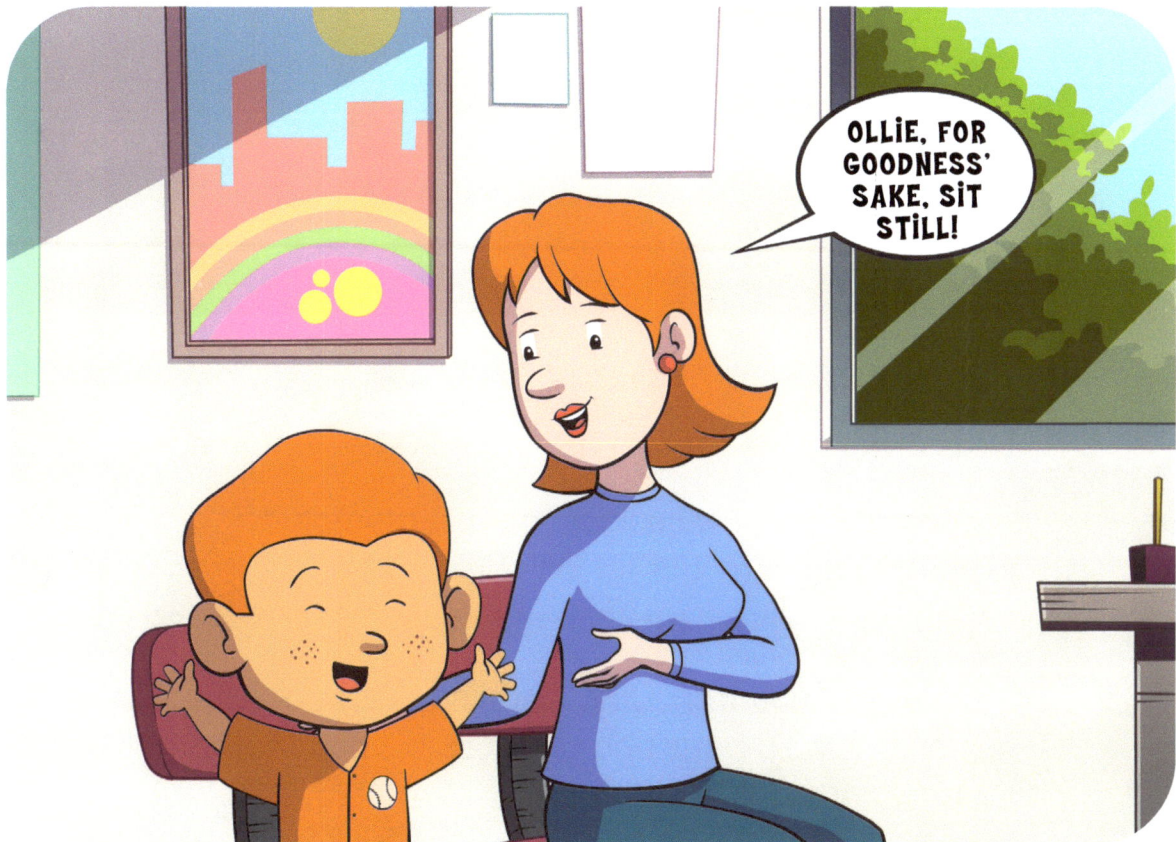

Wait, what? I had been thinking about getting better, not really about risking a reaction. That scared me. No way! Shots? Throwing up? I decided not to risk it.

I slid down in my chair while Nurse Rose went over complicated instructions with my mom.

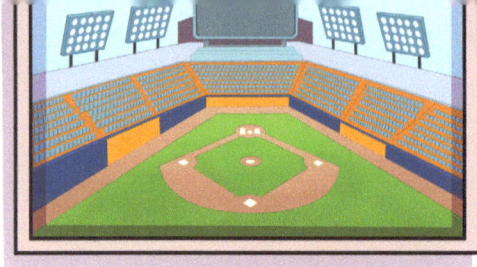

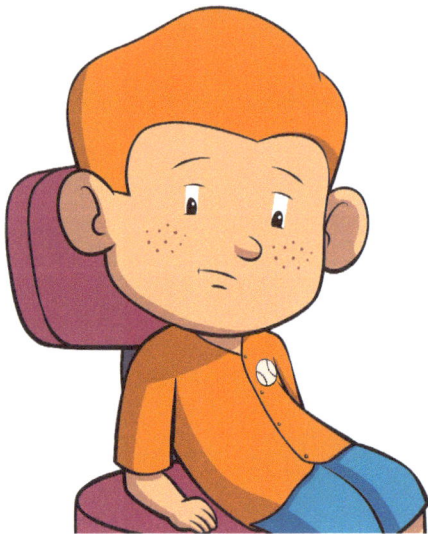

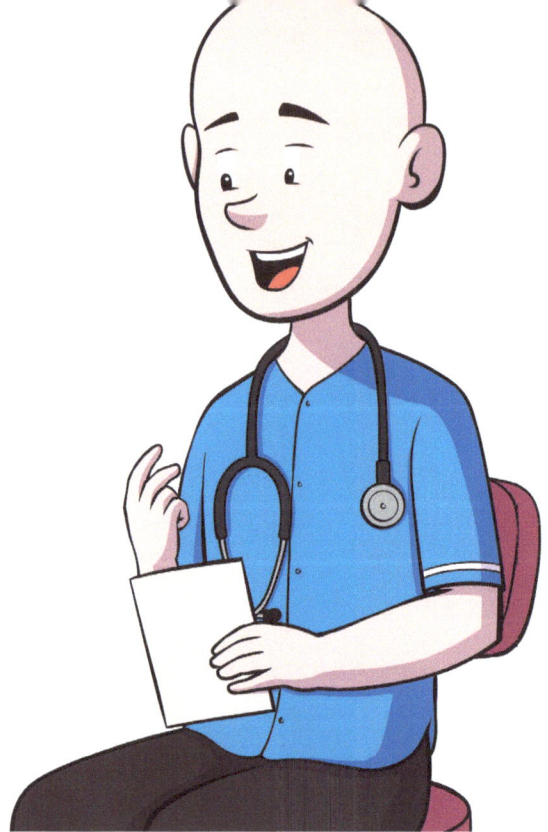

Dr. Browne came back in and sat down next to me.

"I won't do it. I know I said I'd do it," I mumbled, looking at my lap, "but I don't think I want to anymore."

"This will set you free, Ollie. I studied in school for 26 years to help boys and girls just like you," said Dr. Browne.

"Wow, that's a long time! I hate going to school. The teachers are always so careful around me. It's a pain. And some of the other kids are really mean."

"It won't fix everything, but OIT is one thing we can do to help keep you safe at school."

I stared at my shoes. "I'm scared."

"I'm scared of things sometimes too, Ollie," Dr. Browne said, "but I promise this will help, and I'll stay right with you."

"What are you scared of?" I looked up.

"Calling people I don't know on the phone." He smiled, "Actually, I have a call to make today that I've been putting off. Make you a deal, Ollie. You drink that, and I'll go make my call. We can face our fears together."

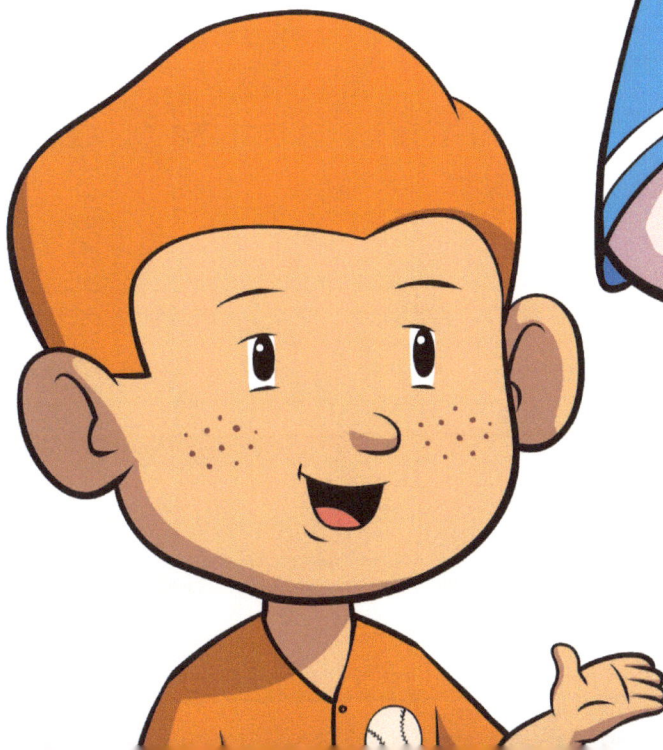

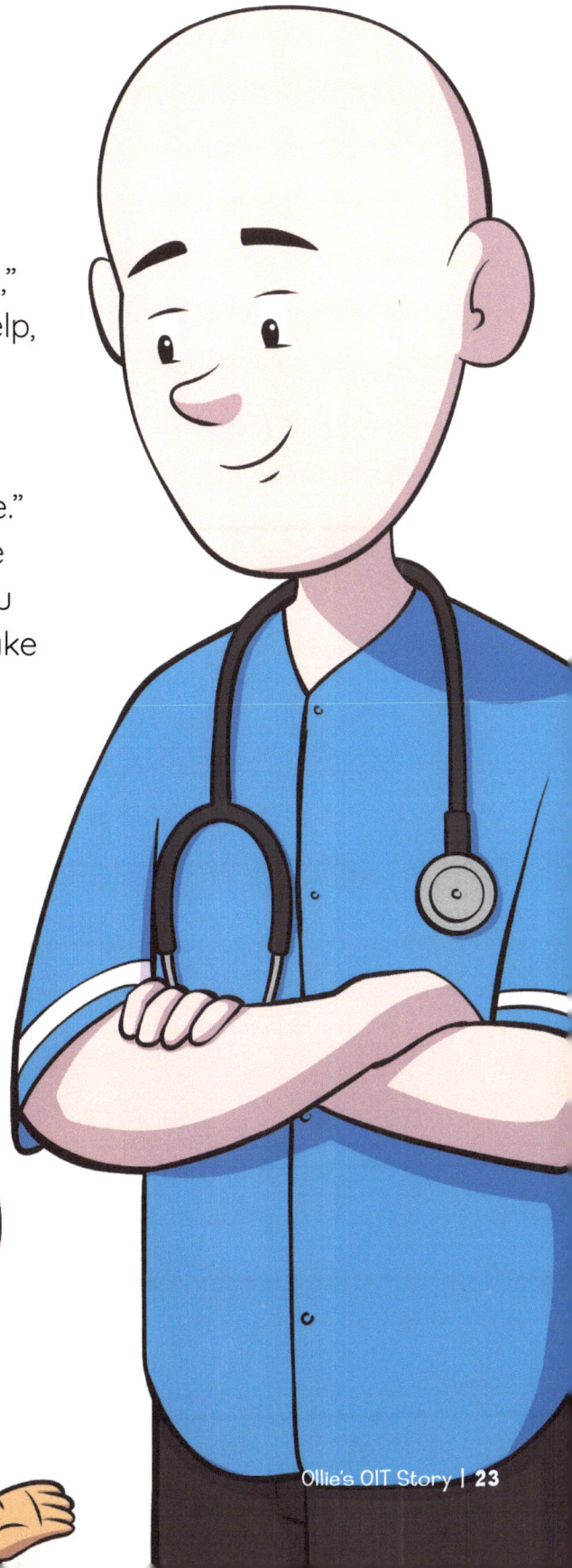

"Okay," I took a deep breath, closed my eyes, and SLURP! It was really sweet.

I waited. I didn't feel funny anywhere.

"Ollie, rest quietly now and we'll check on you. But I think you'll be fine."

"OK, Dr. Browne. Now you go make your phone call!"

"I don't want to," he crossed his arms and pouted. Then he winked at me and went out to make his call.

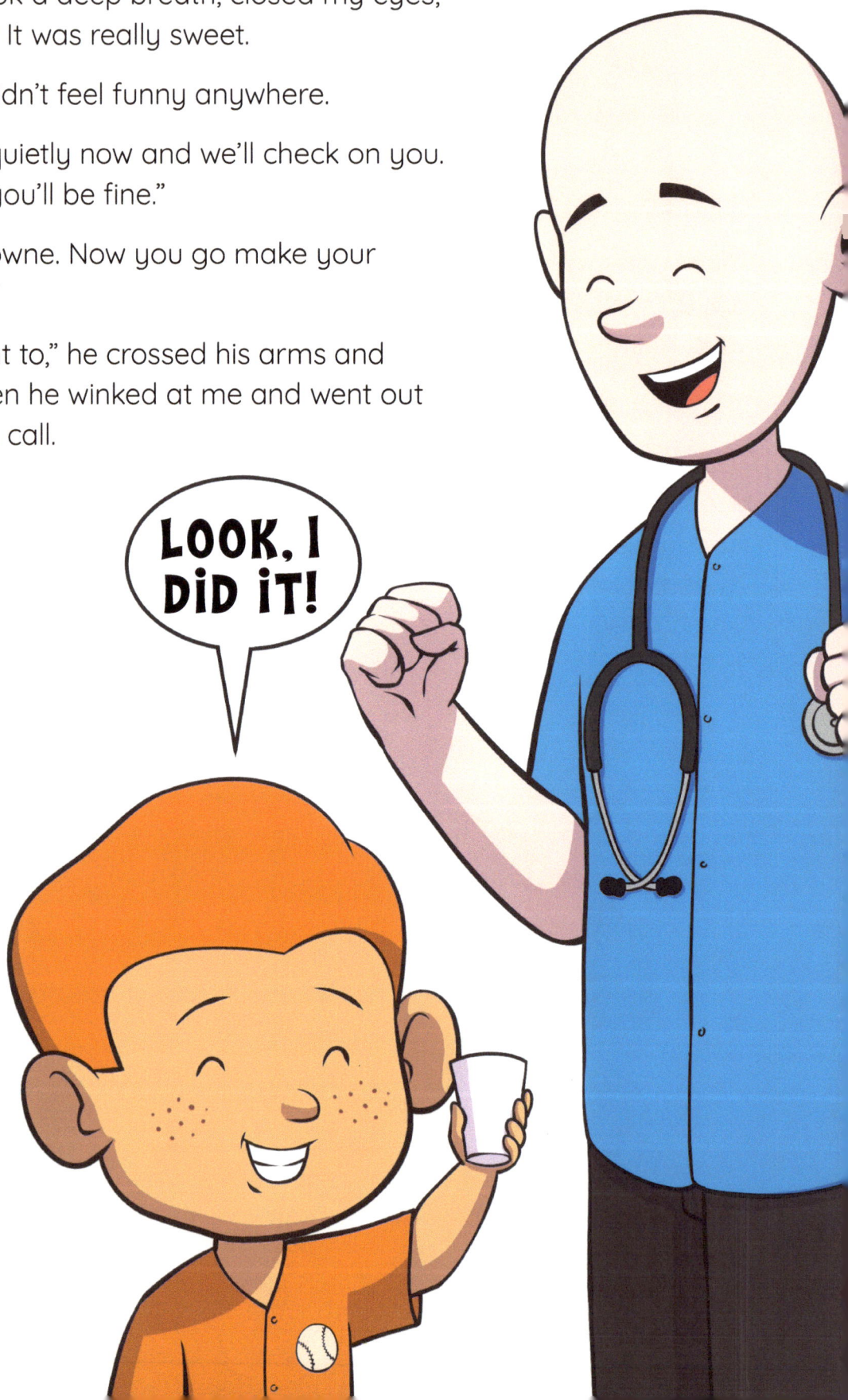

LOOK, I DID IT!

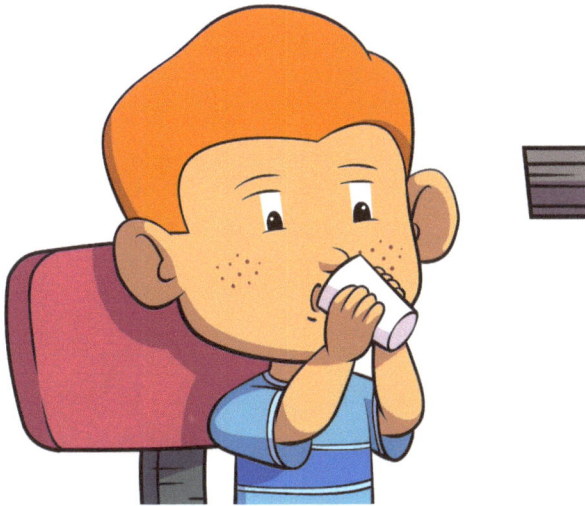

At home, I had to drink a dose of the peanut juice every day. We were always watching to make sure my body didn't react. Mom could text the office if I told her anything felt funny.

Resting after my dose was important so my body could concentrate on dealing with the peanuts. We figured out that I should take it close to bedtime.

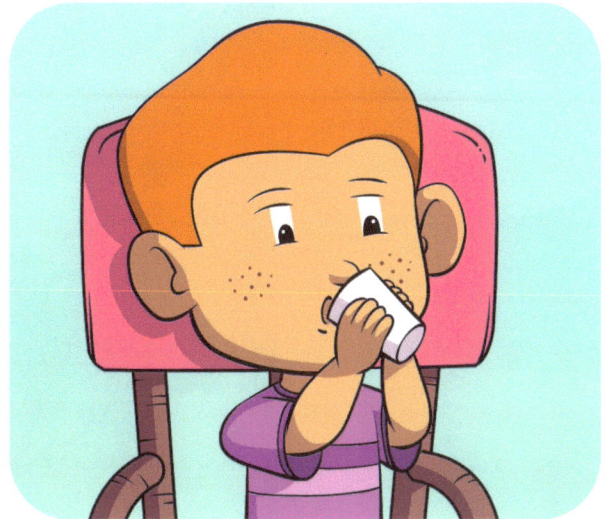

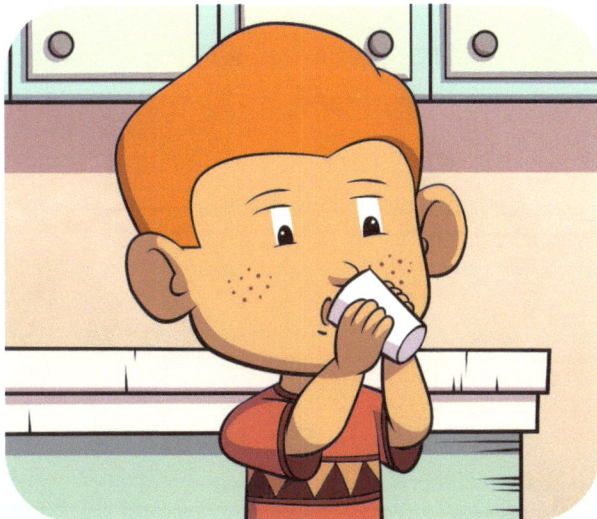

After my dose, I did quiet stuff near Mom for an hour. I'd usually watch a video or play a game.

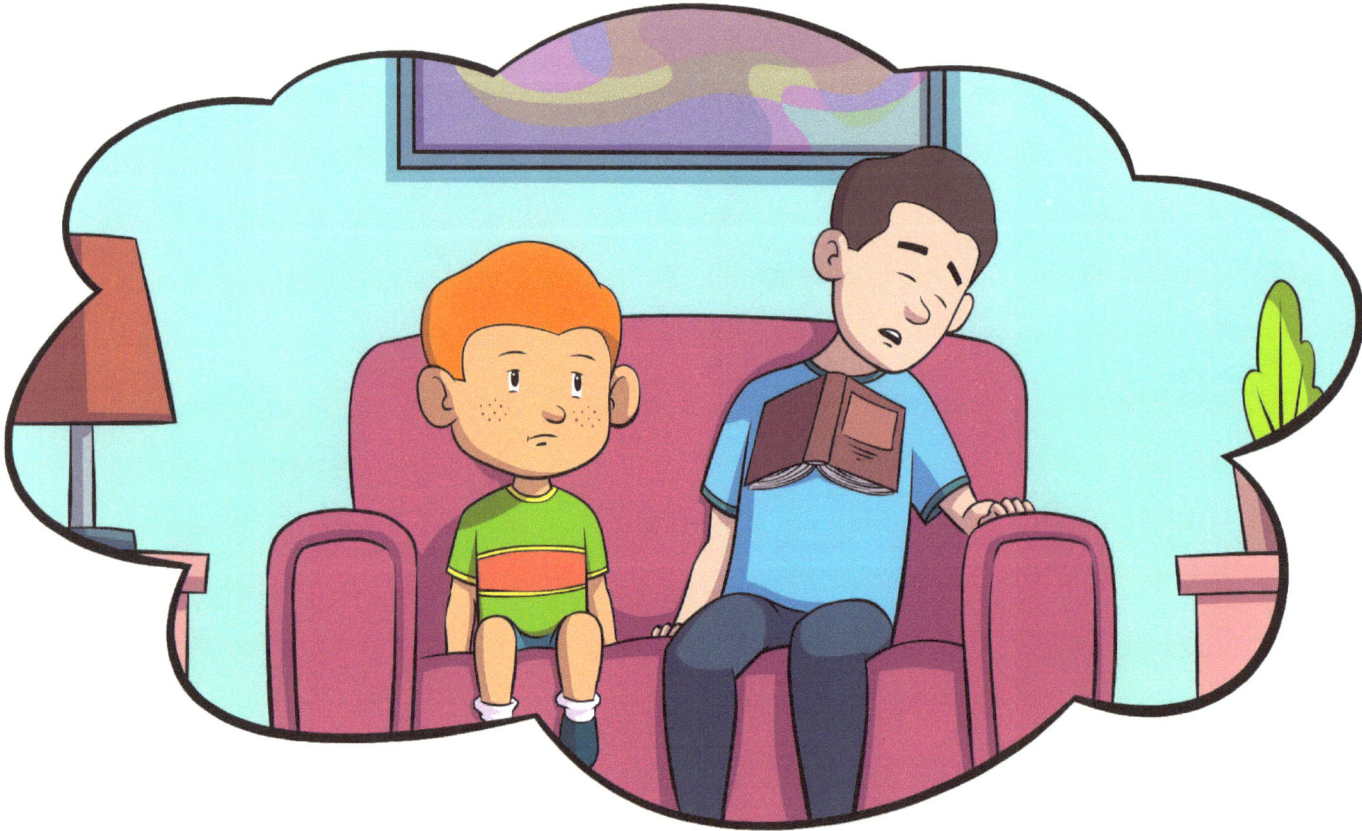

Mom got the idea to stop at the library on our way home from the doctor. If Dad got home before I went to bed, he'd read to me from books we'd picked out— though sometimes he fell asleep before the end.

I had to go to the doctor every week for a long time. Each visit they were adding bigger doses of peanut into my drink.

One day the nurses showed Mom how to measure out a tiny piece of a peanut for me. I was going to actually chew one!

Nurse Rose scooped me a small cup of mint chocolate chip ice cream, explaining that the cold and mint make it hard to taste the peanut. Mom pushed the tiny piece into the ice cream and gave it to me.

"Okay, Ollie. On the count of three, we eat it."

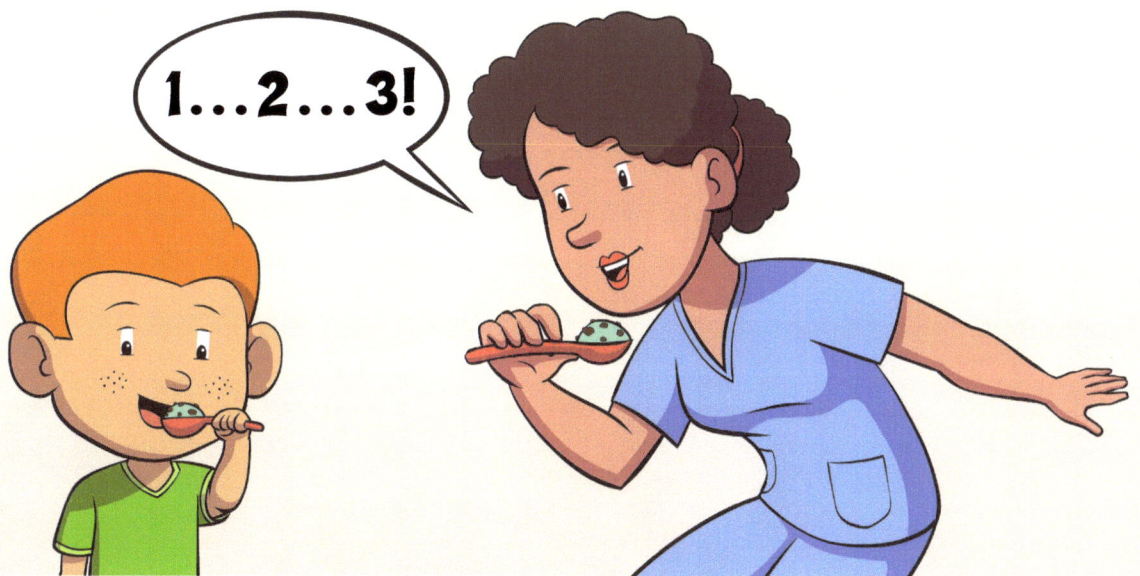

I crunched something. Maybe it was a chocolate chip.

"This is one of the best parts of working here," Nurse Rose said, licking the scoop.

After a few weeks, I was eating a whole peanut every day, even without ice cream.

Finally, Dr. Browne told me that the next week would be my Final Challenge. That sounded very fancy and official, but he said I'd just have to eat a lot of chocolate-covered peanut candies. If all went well, I'd graduate.

That sounded great … if I passed. But what if I had a reaction? What if OIT didn't work on my body after all?

That evening, I didn't read with Dad. We talked and we made our Plan.

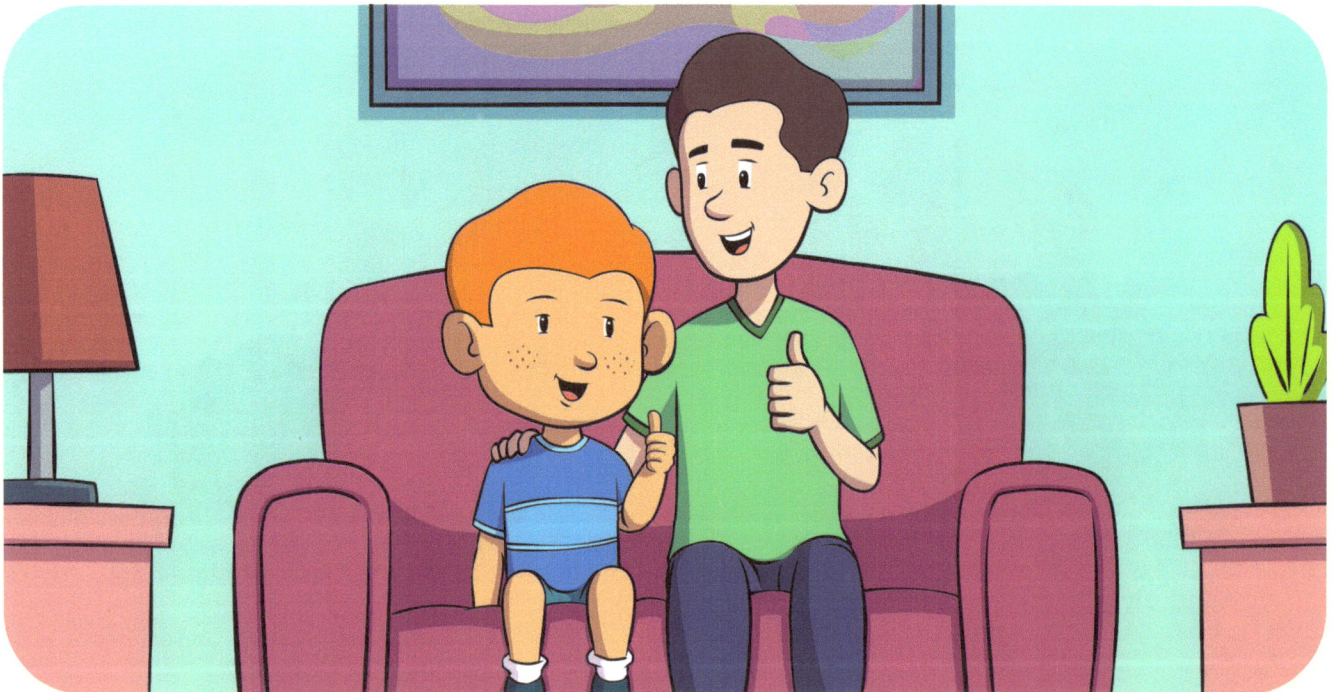

When we got to Dr. Browne's office, Mom counted out a huge pile of chocolate-covered peanut candies.

I took a deep breath and started the Plan.

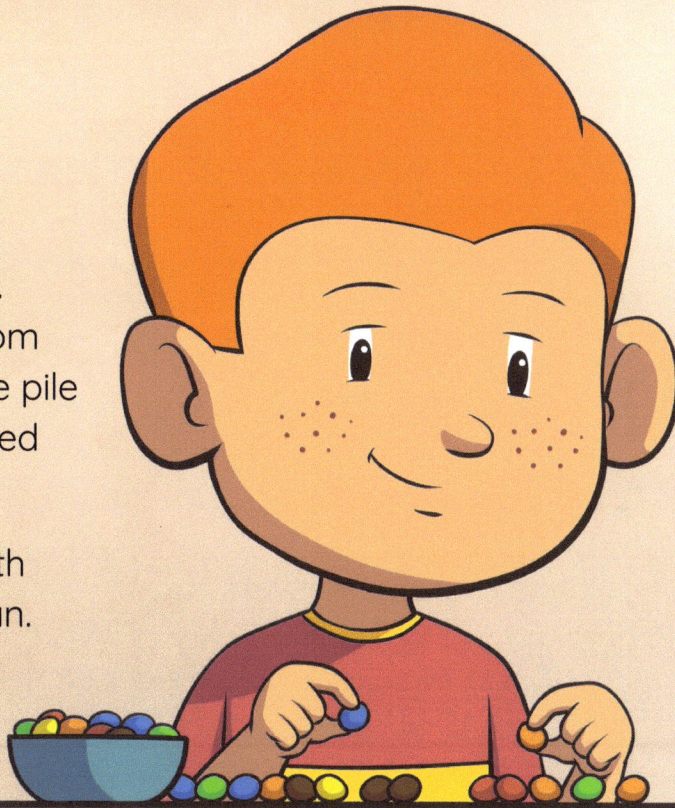

I ate all the greens. "Green for go," I said.

I ate the blue ones next. There were exactly seven of them, and I'm seven. They tasted so good.

I ate the yellow ones next because I'm a yellow belt in tae kwon do now.

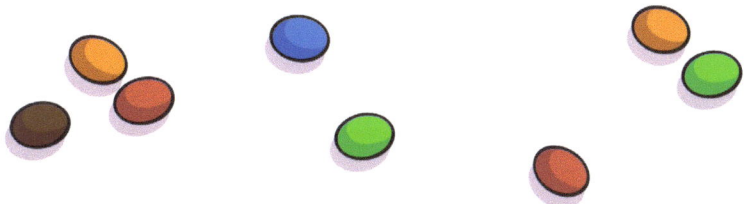

Then I said, "Roses are red. I'll eat these for you, Nurse Rose!"

I chewed for a long time before I could say, "These brown ones are for Dr. Browne."

There were only the orange ones left now, just as Dad and I had planned.

"Mom, if I'm fine, can we go to a baseball game soon?"

She told me not to talk with my mouth full, but she smiled. "Maybe we will!"

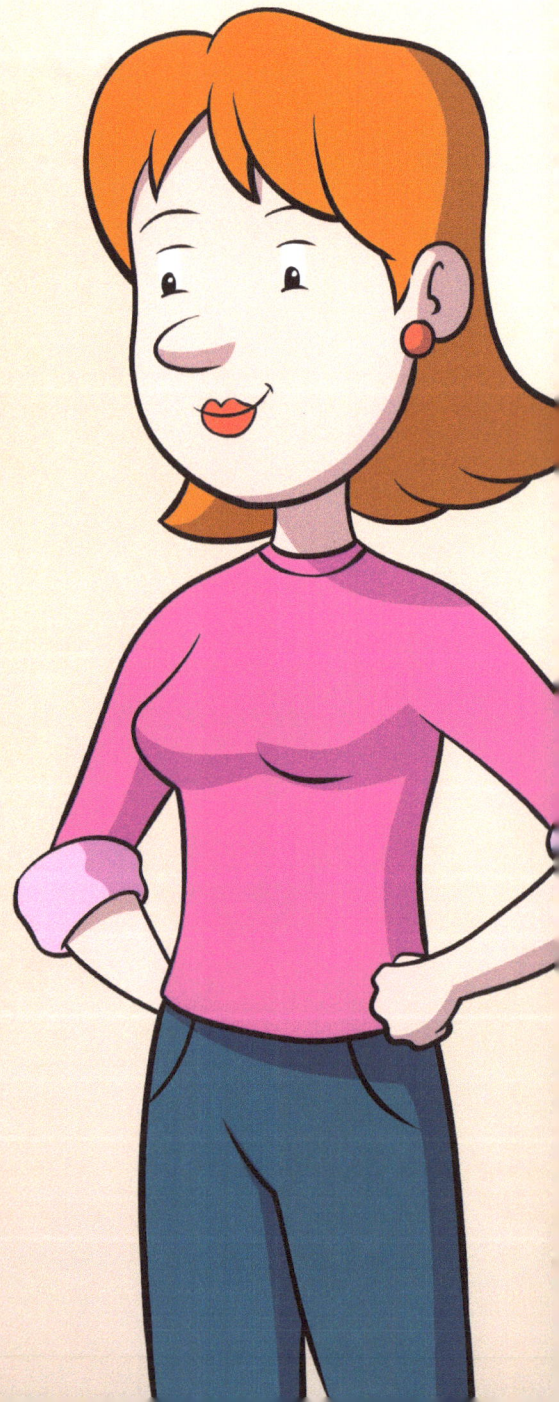

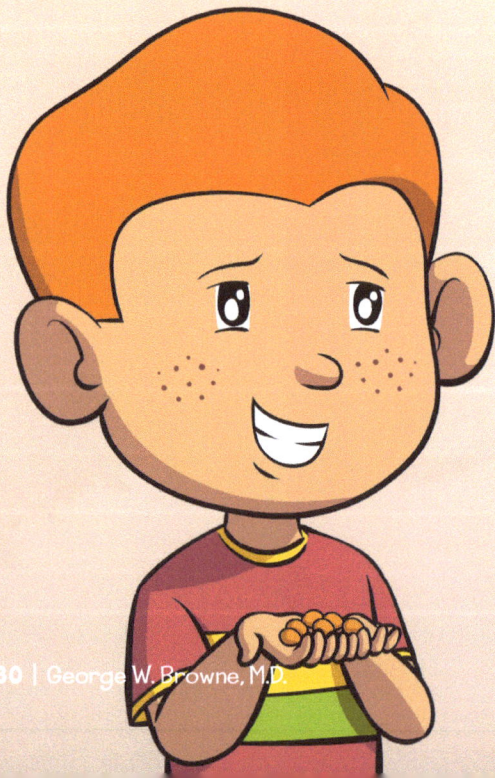

We had to wait and see what my body would do. I was full of candy and pretty excited—and a little nervous.

Nurse Rose came back to check on me with Dr. Browne. I had to tell them that my stomach felt kind of weird, but they checked me all over and didn't think it was a reaction. Mom had my emergency shots with her (she still has to have them handy for me, just in case).

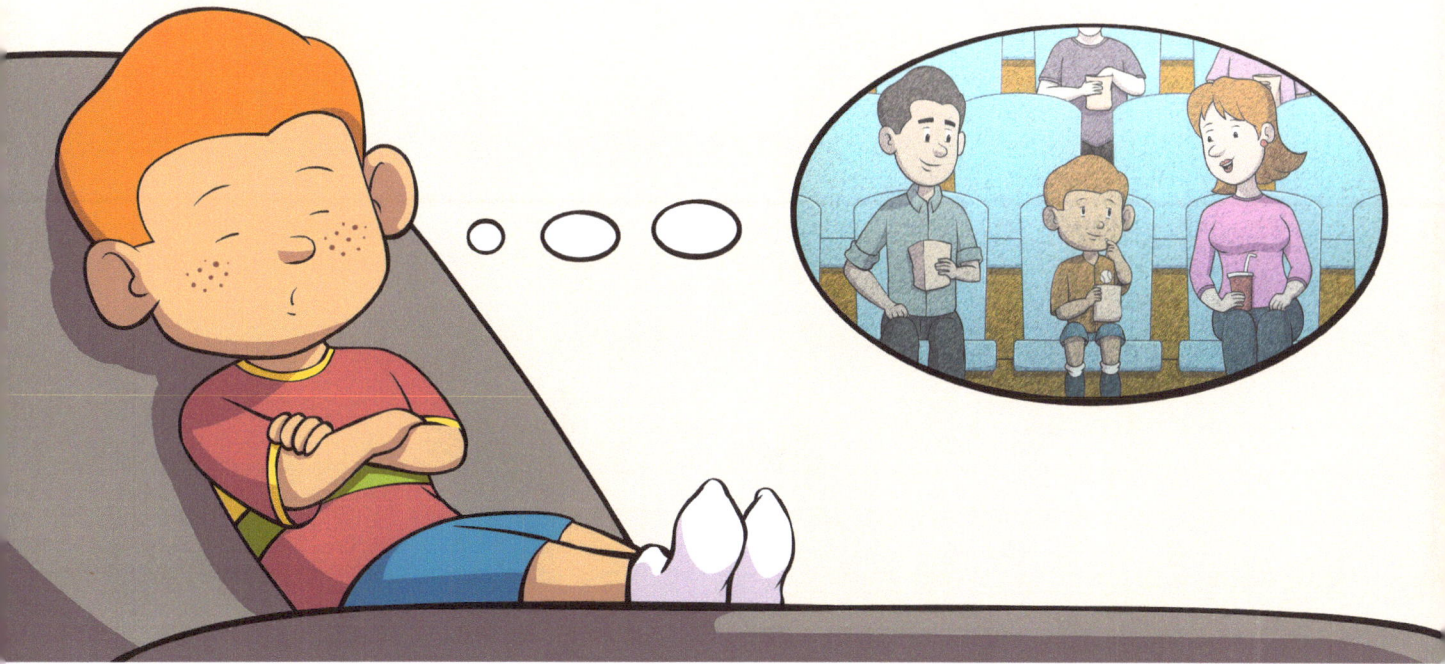

I closed my eyes. If I passed this test, I'd be done! I could eat peanuts anytime, anywhere I wanted to. I'd still have to be careful and let my body rest if I did, and eat eight peanuts every day to keep my body used to them. But that'd be so much better than living scared.

I wouldn't have to sit alone at my special lunch table at school. No one could tease me about peanut butter. But the bullies had left me alone since my mom and their moms became friends.

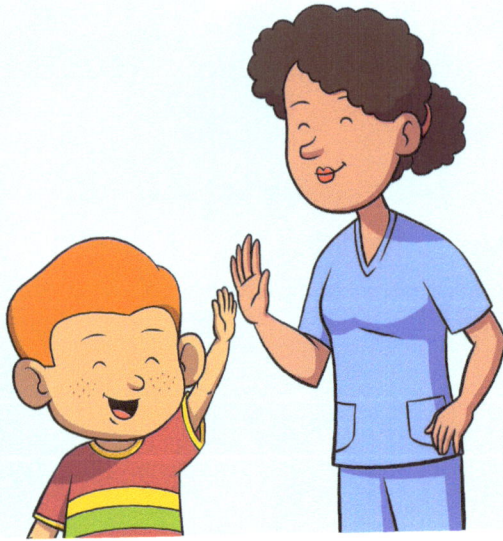

"Ollie, how are you feeling?" Nurse Rose asked as she walked back into the room.

"Fine!" I said, sitting up straight. "Is the time up? Did I pass?"

"Yes!"

I yelled and we high-fived.

Suddenly, Nurse Rose rang a cowbell. All the staff came pouring in, clapping.

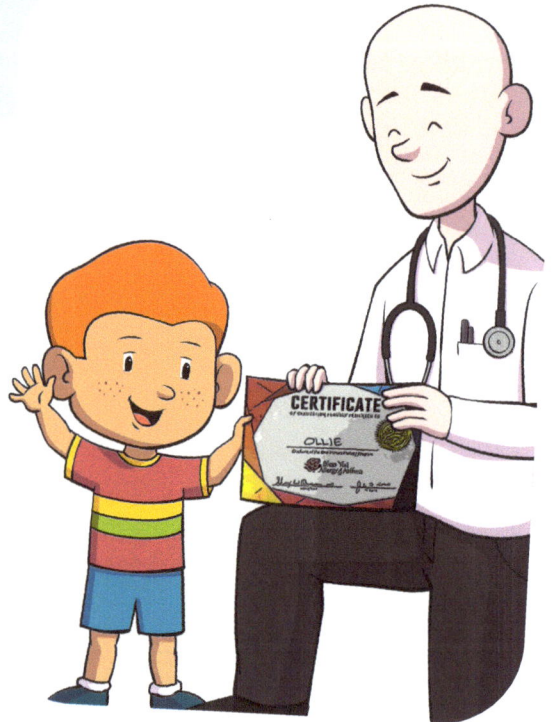

Someone handed me a certificate and took my picture to put on the Wall of Fame. My dad walked in holding Ethan. "Surprise!" he yelled, as I ran over for a hug.

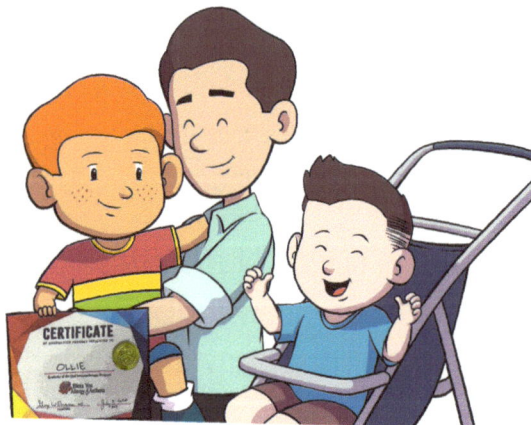

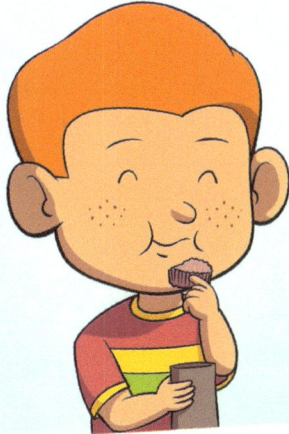

Dr. Browne handed me a giant peanut butter cup and shook my hand. I opened it and broke off two pieces. I handed one to him and another to Dad.

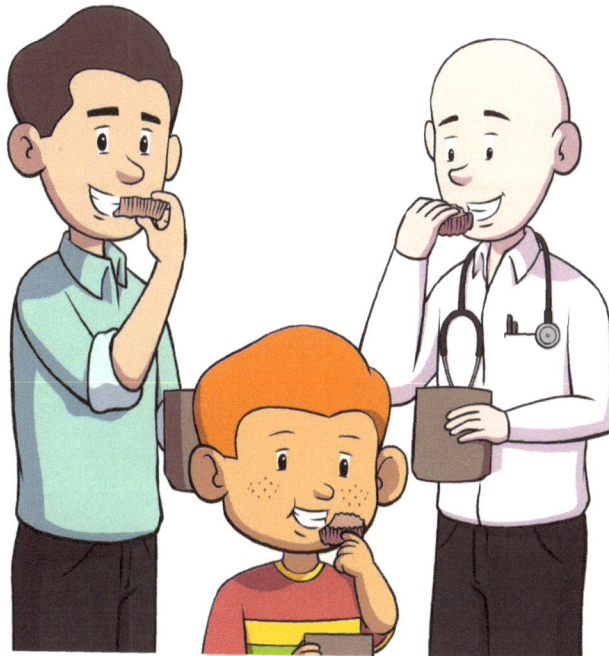

"1 . . . 2 . . . 3!" We popped our pieces into our mouths.

And tasted.

And smiled.

It was so good!

Everyone was laughing and talking. My smile was so big that my face started to hurt.

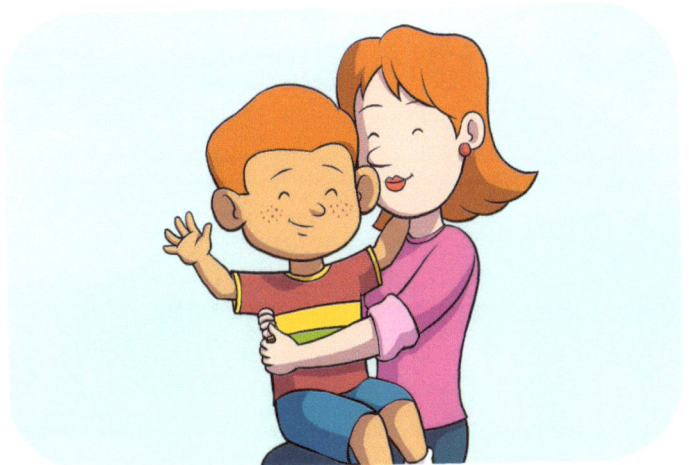

So, that's my OIT story. It's really cool to be the one sharing my story at an OIT information night. I thought I'd be really scared to talk in front of you all, but after facing my peanut allergy, I guess I've gotten braver.

I hope you like the slideshow we made. Some of the pictures are pretty funny. I hope your family decides to do OIT too. It is so worth it.

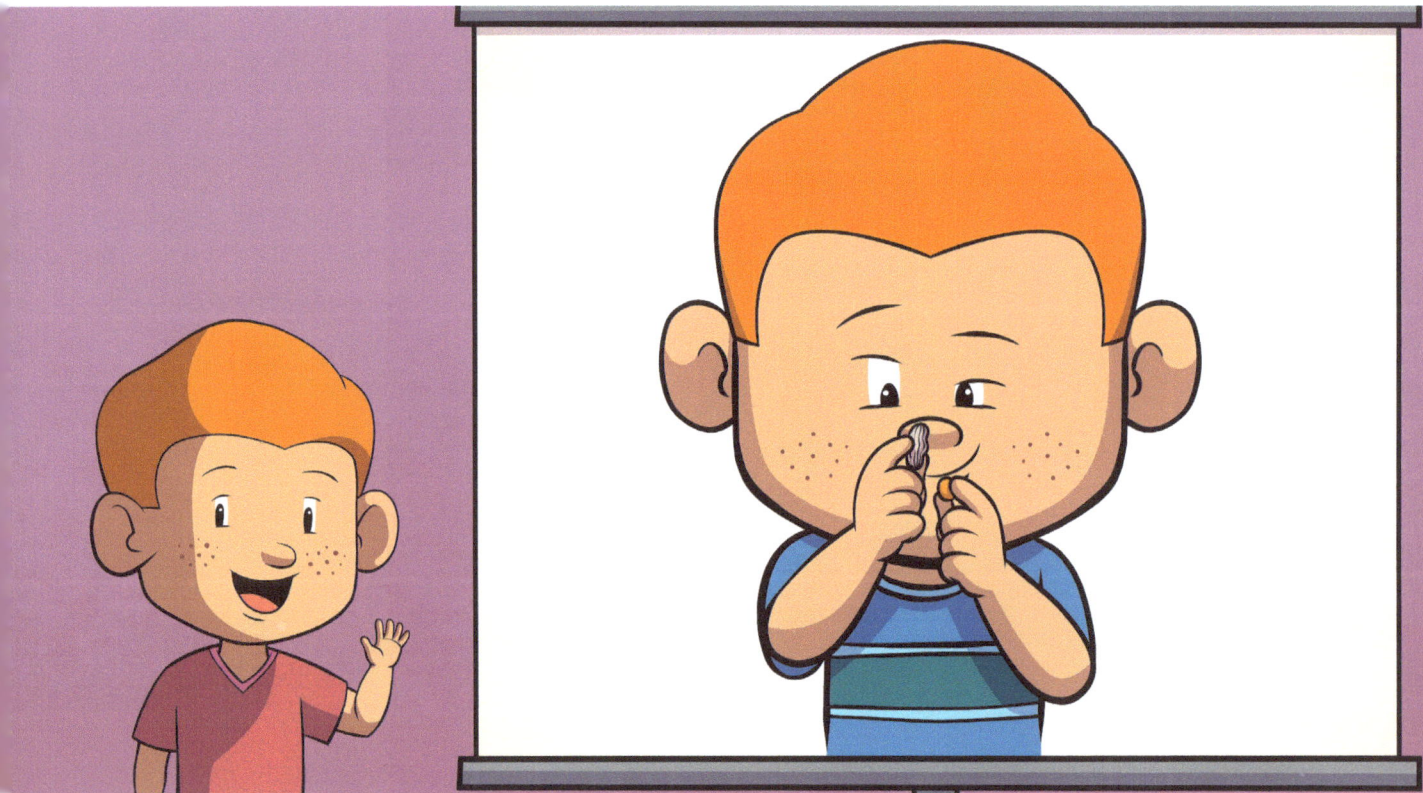

Oh, and guess what?

This Saturday, Dad is taking me to the baseball game!

DEAR MOMS AND DADS,

Hello, my name is Dr. George Browne. I hope you enjoyed following Ollie's journey through oral immunotherapy (OIT), which was inspired by so many real kids and families I have had the privilege to help every day at Bless You Allergy & Asthma.

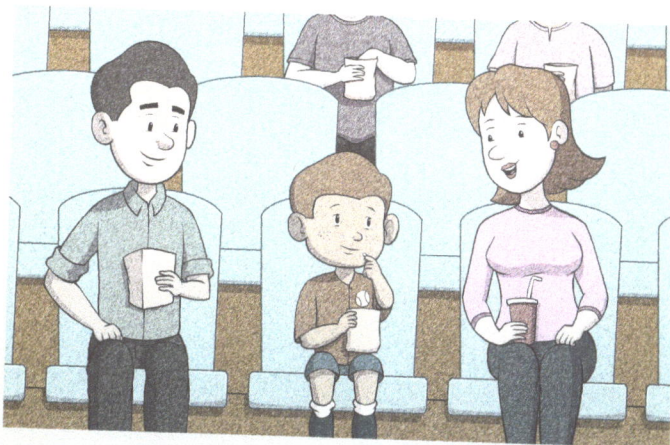

In addition to being a board-certified allergist and immunologist, I'm a dad. My wife, Jennifer, and I have seven awesome and active kids. Two of them have dealt with food allergies. I know all about the restaurant limitations, the label reading, the expensive substitute foods, the making two different versions of things, the fear when they experience a reaction, the pain of watching them feel different or left out . . . it's hard. Really hard!

My early experience as an allergist was equally frustrating. There was little substantial help I could offer beyond running tests to determine which foods to avoid. It fell so short of what I wanted for those families, especially since I knew full well that 40% of these folks would experience a life-threatening accidental ingestion.

When I learned about Dr. Wasserman's successful work developing OIT, I contacted him immediately and asked if he would teach me. It is an absolute privilege to carry his area of expertise back to my patients. I am honored to walk alongside families as they face their fears head-on and help them journey to a safe place. Our staff at Bless You Allergy & Asthma loves to celebrate the victories each family has as they make their lives better through OIT.

Food Allergy Conqueror: Ollie's OIT Story has been a labor of love between my wife and me over the last year. Her passion for teaching children led me to see the importance of writing a picture book to help explain the OIT process to our young patients. I hope Ollie will be a friend and inspiration for them. I hope this book gives them the words and understanding they need to own the process for themselves and to share what they are going through with others.

Having food allergies does not have to be a life sentence. OIT is an option. If you live in the Houston area, call today and let's change the trajectory of your life for the better. I can't wait to meet you!

My very best,

George W. Browne, M.D., FAAAAI, FACAAI
Board-Certified Allergist and Immunologist

P.S. If you have a friend or loved one living with food allergies, please pass along a copy of *Food Allergy Conqueror: Ollie's OIT Story* to them!

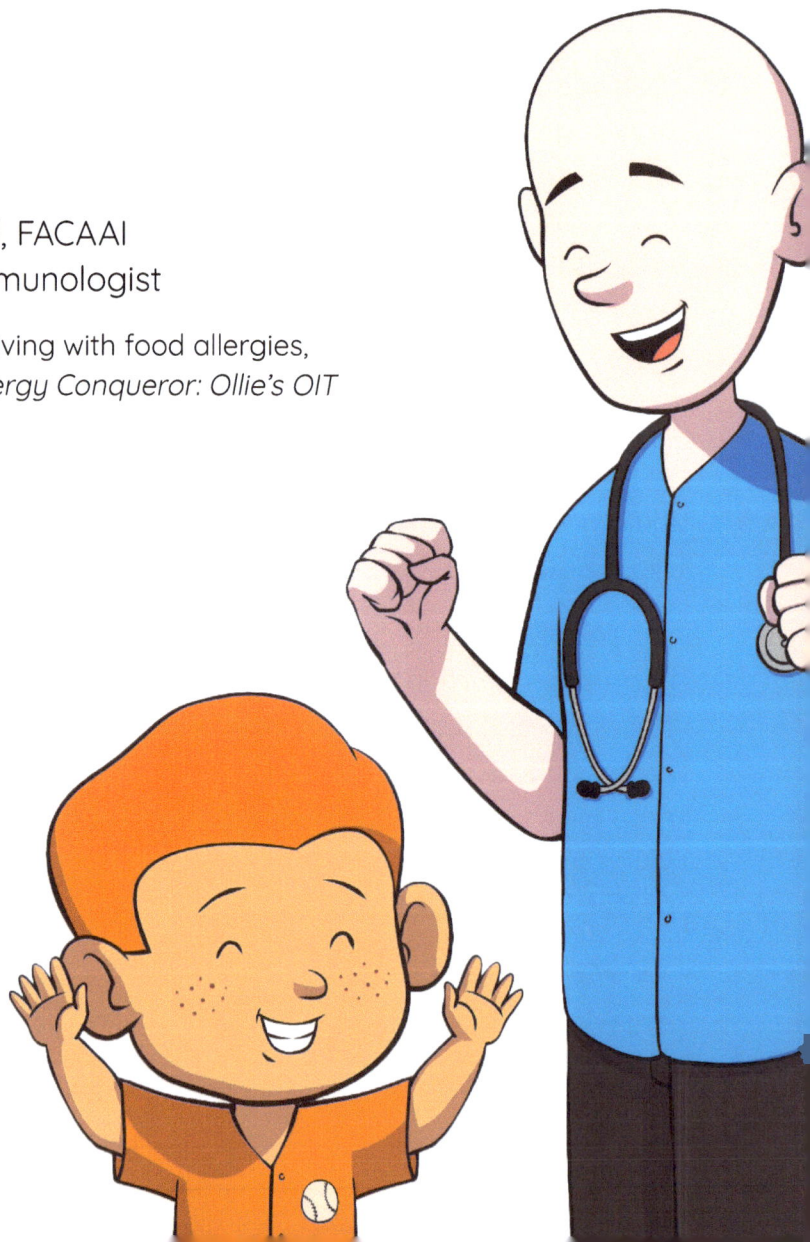

ABOUT THE AUTHORS

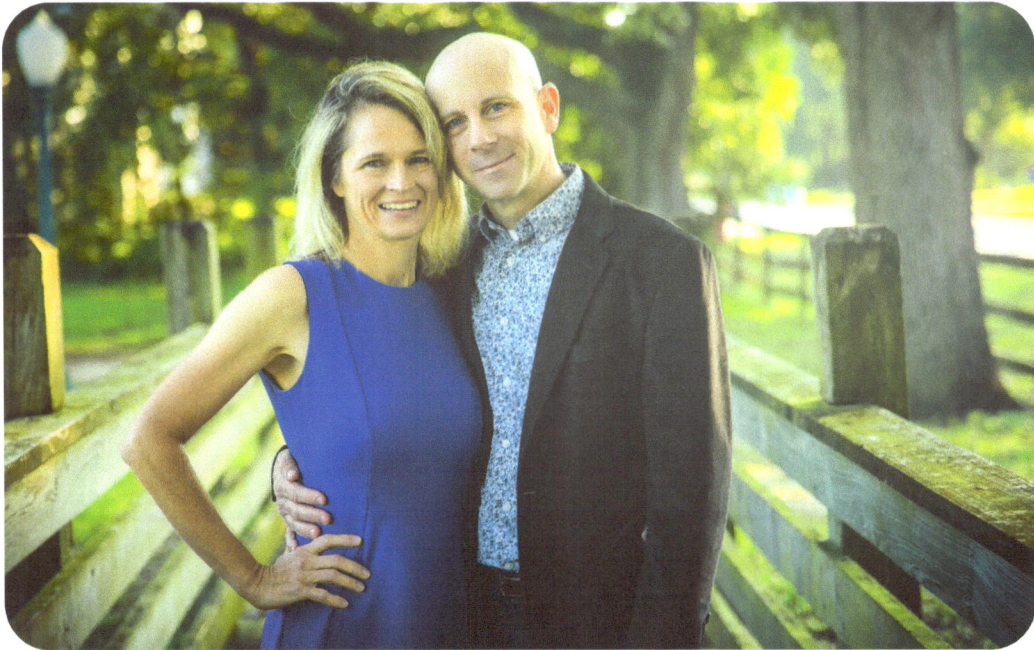

GEORGE W. BROWNE, M.D., FAAAAI, FACAAI, is a board-certified allergist and immunologist. He has wanted to help and heal children since he was in the 7th grade. After many years of training, he is thrilled to be running the Bless You Allergy & Asthma clinics in the Houston area. Changing the trajectory of a child's life and freeing them from the fear associated with food allergy through OIT has become one of the most fulfilling parts of his work. When not in clinic, Dr. Browne is most likely watching a soccer game, eating a chocolate chip cookie, or enjoying time with his wife and seven children. And, as often as possible, doing all of them at once!

JENNIFER BROWNE is blessed to be married to Dr. Browne and mother to their seven amazing children. As a childhood development specialist and lifelong book lover, she developed a passion to get *Food Allergy Conqueror: Ollie's OIT Story* into print to give children a vehicle to help them understand and be able to share with others the OIT journey. Her other passions include God, making homeschooling fun, fitness, and vanilla ice cream cones with rainbow sprinkles.

OIT RESOURCES

What is OIT?

OIT is short for oral immunotherapy, a treatment guided by a board-certified allergist to free the patient from the fear and danger of accidental ingestion and to allow the patient to freely eat the problem food without negative effect. Basically, it is a gradual retraining of the immune system to tolerate the food allergens by regular ingesting of small samples of the allergic food.

Is OIT effective?

Over 80% of the patients who complete OIT treatment experience successful results: Safety from food allergies, freedom from a lifestyle of constant vigilance, and the ability to eat the food that once threatened their well-being.

Is OIT safe?

Yes. Under the watchful eye of a specially trained physician, any reactions your body may experience will be anticipated and prepared for. Epinephrine would be administered immediately and your rate of desensitization slowed or paused as needed. Compare this to the scary statistics that 50–75% of food-allergic patients experience an accidental ingestion that causes a meaningful reaction during their lifetime and may not have the personnel or equipment near them to deal with the crisis.

Is OIT new? Why haven't I heard about this before?

The science behind OIT dates back to attempts in the Middle Ages to develop tolerances to poison. More popular today are allergy shots, which have been using the same technique to successfully deal with environmental allergies for over 100 years. Serious clinical studies on the effectiveness of OIT are more recent, and very promising. Over the last 10 years, both the continuing studies and the experience of clinical practices confirm an over 80% success rate for OIT.

Is OIT really legit?

Yes. Here are some of the professional organizations that have commented positively on the clinical trials being done to study the effectiveness of OIT:

- The American Academy of Pediatrics[1]
- National Institutes of Health[2]
- American Academy of Allergy and Immunology[3]
- Acta Paediatrica[4]

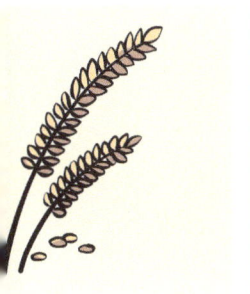

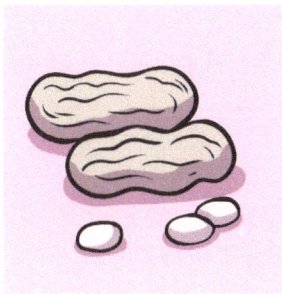

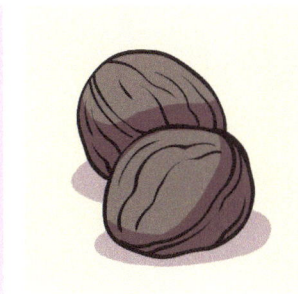

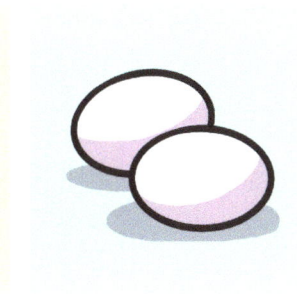

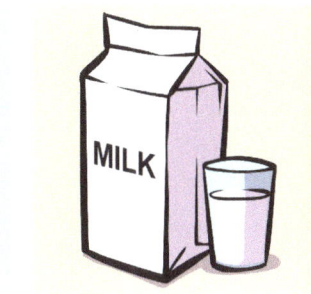

How long does OIT treatment take?

Usually between 6 and 12 months. It is an investment of time, but one with results that last a lifetime.

Who pays for OIT treatment?

Depending on your plan, your insurance should cover this treatment. We find over 85% of our patients do have insurance coverage for OIT.

Has the FDA approved OIT treatment?

OIT involves no prescription, just the gradual supervised increase of tolerance to food, so it is outside the FDA's jurisdiction. Please do not wait for an approval that will never come, because it cannot.

Can I try this myself at home?

No. OIT is a medical treatment and should only be performed under the close supervision of a trained medical professional.

Where can I go to learn more?

Please visit our website, BlessYouAllergy.com, for more information about OIT. We also recommend the following resources:

- *The Food Allergy Fix* by Sakina Shikari Bajowala, M.D.
- www.OITworks.org
- www.OIT101.org

If you live nearby, please make an appointment.
We can't wait to meet you!

[1] https://onlinelibrary.wiley.com/doi/abs/10.1111/apa.13251
[2] https://www.jacionline.org/article/S0091-6749(16)30531-0/fulltext
[3] https://www.jacionline.org/article/S0091-6749(16)00117-2/fulltext
[4] https://onlinelibrary.wiley.com/doi/abs/10.1111/apa.13251

ABOUT BLESS YOU ALLERGY & ASTHMA

Our mission is to make our patients' lives better by caring for their allergy and asthma issues with the most effective treatments available, while at the same time providing an unparalleled patient-provider relationship. We seek always to provide exceptional care while bringing joy and reverencing the profound dignity of each unique person. Our team of highly trained experts feels blessed to be able to work together in this unique clinic. We operate as a peaceful, joyful unit, and we look forward to welcoming your family into this atmosphere.

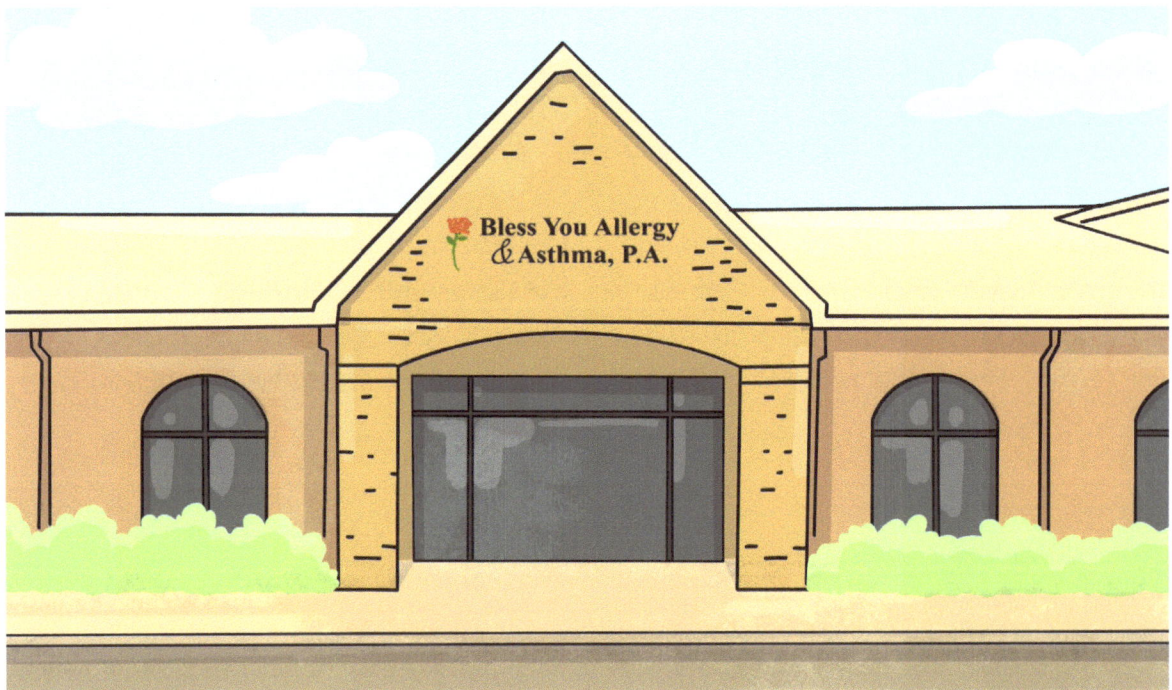

Please call today to make your appointment at one of our Houston-area clinics!

FRIENDSWOOD, TX (281) 648-1025 | **CYPRESS, TX** (281) 213-2522

"Children are not a distraction from more important work. They are the most important work."

—C.S. Lewis

www.ingramcontent.com/pod-product-compliance
Lightning Source LLC
Chambersburg PA
CBHW060833270326
41933CB00002B/76